MEDICAL
INTELLIGENCE
UNIT

# GRAFT-VERSUS-HOST DISEASE

## Nelson J. Chao, M.D.

Bone Marrow Transplantation Program
Stanford University Medical Center

R.G. LANDES COMPANY
AUSTIN

MEDICAL INTELLIGENCE UNIT
GRAFT-VERSUS-HOST DISEASE: PAST, PRESENT AND FUTURE
R.G. LANDES COMPANY
Austin

CRC Press is the exclusive worldwide distributor of publications
of the Medical Intelligence Unit.
CRC Press, 2000 Corporate Blvd., NW, Boca Raton, FL 33431. Phone: 407/994-0555.

Submitted: February 1994

Published: April 1994

Production Manager: Terry Nelson
Copy Editor: Karen Ross

Please address all inquiries to the Publisher:
R.G. Landes Company, 909 Pine Street, Georgetown, TX 78626
or
P.O. Box 4858, Austin, TX 78765

Phone: 512/ 863 7762; FAX: 512/ 863 0081

ISBN 1-57059-129-6
CATALOG # LN9129

While the authors, editors and publisher believe that drug selection and dosage and the specifications and usage of equipment and devices, as set forth in this book, are in accord with current recommendations and practice at the time of publication, they make no warranty, expressed or implied, with respect to material described in this book. In view of the ongoing research, equipment development, changes in governmental regulations and the rapid accumulation of information relating to the biomedical sciences, the reader is urged to carefully review and evaluate the information provided herein.

Library of Congress Cataloging-in-Publication Data

Chao, Nelson J.
    Graft-versus-host disease / Nelson J. Chao.
        p. cm.—(Medical intelligence unit)
    Includes bibliographical references and index.
    ISBN 1-57059-129-6
    1. Graft versus host disease. I. Title. II. Series.
    [DLNM: 1. Graft vs Host Disease. 2. Transplantation—adverse effects. WO 680 G461g
1994]
R123.5.C48 1994
617.9'5—dc20
DNLM/DLC
for Library of Congress
                                                    94-14221
                                                    CIP

## DEDICATION

This book is dedicated to the patients and their families whose courage laid the foundation for a successful treatment modality.

# CONTENTS

# ACKNOWLEDGMENTS

I would like to thank my parents for the past direction, my wife, Norma for her continued efforts and patience, and my mentor Karl G. Blume for his gentle (and sometimes not so gentle) guidance. I would also like to thank my collegues at Stanford, Robert S. Negrin, Gwynn D. Long, Paul G. Schlegel, Rina Aharoni, Dawn E. Smilek and Hugh O. McDevitt for the many, many stimulating discussions. Finally I am indebted to Marsha Roon for her editorial skills and to Sara E. Clark for her expert secretarial assistance. Whatever mistakes are found are mine and mine only.

# CHAPTER 1

# HISTORICAL PERSPECTIVE

## INTRODUCTION

Graft-versus-host disease (GVHD) is the result of an intricate response found in our immune system. There is no other clinical situation that stresses the importance of being histocompatible. As individuals evolved from single cell organisms, there arose the need to distinguish those cells that were part of the "self" from those that were "non-self"—presumably because of the need to destroy foreign invaders to ensure survival. In more highly developed beings, this distinction between self and non-self is made out by specialized cells of the immune system. With the advent of modern medicine and the ability and desire to treat difficult diseases, foreign cells (blood, organs and bone marrow) have been transplanted in an attempt to save patients. Mixing foreign donor cells with the patient's own cells can result in graft-versus-host reaction and GVHD. This disease process is similar to the reaction seen in experimental models.

Graft-versus-host reaction was first observed in the early 20th century by James B. Murphy, who was interested in studying cancer. In his investigations, Murphy grafted normal tissue onto the chorioallantoic membrane of seven-day chicken eggs as controls for tumor cell implantation. When these eggs were grafted with certain normal tissues and were opened later, there were scattered whitish nodules around the area of implantation.[1] There was also splenic enlargement with nodules similar to those observed at the implantation site, and occasionally nodules were found in the embryonic skin. Murphy also made the observation that these changes were frequently found after splenic implantation, more irregularly after liver implantation; rarely after kidney, and not at all after muscle or cartilage implantation. These observations were made decades prior to the discovery of lymphocytes and graft-versus-host reaction. Initially, the nodules and the splenic enlargement were attributed to some type of stimulatory factor.

It would be logical to assume that the concept of GVHD arose from experimental bone marrow transplantation (BMT). However, this assumption is not correct. The suggestion of GVHD arose from kidney transplantation in dogs. Simonsen demonstrated that the rejection of a second kidney from a given donor to the same recipient led to an accelerated rate of rejection.[2] Histological sections of the rejected kidneys demonstrated an interstitial infiltrate with small lymphocytes and larger pyrioninophylic cells. Although the origin of these cells was not readily apparent, there arose the novel idea that the local pyrioninophylic reaction could be specifically directed against the allogeneic antigens of the host.[3]

The demonstration of true GVHD owes much to the study of immunological tolerance. Billingham, Brent and Medawar were interested in inducing embryonic tolerance in chicken skin homografts by using adult homologous blood.[4,5] To their dismay, about 95% of the recipients died just before hatching. These investigators observed that embryonic blood was innocuous, that adult homologous blood failed to harm newly hatched chicks, and that adult duck blood was usually inoffensive, suggesting that death was not caused by infection. The high mortality rate was seen only when the adult homologous blood was combined with the chick embryos. These observations again led to the possibility that, in the early stages of homograft reaction, immunologically competent cells cause the response against the alien transplantation antigens of the host. Subsequent demonstration that normal peripheral blood contain immunologically competent cells suggested that the pyrioninophylic cells within the homografts were indeed of host origin.[6]

Gowans et al, by inoculating labeled small lymphocytes from parental strain rat donors into F1 hybrids and lethally irradiated mice, confirmed previous indirect evidence that these cells "home" into the lymphoid tissues of the host.[7] Within 24 hours of injection, the cells transformed into large pyrioninophylic cells and responded to stimulation by the foreign antigen of the host. They then underwent rapid division to produce lymphocytes of progressively smaller sizes. These cells also appeared in the lymph nodes of animals undergoing graft-versus-host reactions. This led to the conclusion that a common underlying immunological mechanism is involved.

From these observations, Billingham's work, published as a Harvey lecture in 1966, identified the general criteria necessary for graft-versus-host reactions.[8]

1.  The graft must contain immunologically competent cells.
2.  The host must possess important transplantation isoantigens that are lacking in the graft donor, so that the host appears foreign to it and is therefore capable of stimulating it antigenically.
3.  The host itself must be incapable of mounting an effective immunological reaction against the graft, at least for sufficient time for the latter to manifest its immunological capabilities, i.e., the graft must have some security of tenure.

The description of the GVHD literature in Billingham's original article is an excellent historical review as to what had happened in the field up to that point.

## HISTOLOGICAL CHANGES

The clinical picture in a rodent model with GVHD (formerly known as runt disease) is thickening and subsequent loss of elasticity of the skin, usually accompanied by erythema of the soles of the feet or the skin of the ears. The rigidity of the skin results in the difficulty with gait observed in these animals. There are areas of epidermal cell loss around the ears and nose, as well as near the anus. These areas extend from such sites to involve the whole integument. There is an abrupt cessation of weight gain and many individuals may lose a significant amount of weight. Death usually takes place following loss of 25-30% of their weight. During the terminal phase of this disease, the animals frequently develop diarrhea. A small number, however, develop a chronic form of this runting disease and, occasionally, some animals recover.

Histologically, the skin displays very characteristic and striking abnormalities. There is an infiltration of histocytes with fibroblast proliferation along the dermis. The superficial epidermis becomes abnormally thick with hyperkeratosis and prominent changes in the Malpighian layer. The hair follicles, as well as the sebaceous glands, are also affected. In severe cases, there is disruption of the dermal-epidermal junction. This striking dermatitis is diagnostic of GVHD or runt disease when major histocompatibility complex (MHC) mismatched host and donor combinations are tested. However, this is not an invariable result in all mice strains, specifically when MHC congenic strains are tested.

Two possibilities existed for this dermatitis. It could have been (1) a nonspecific consequence from derangement of the normal host physiology or metabolism or (2) a consequence of a specific reaction on the part of the immunologic competent cells directed against the hosts' skin. To address these two possibilities, Billingham et al transplanted neonatal host rats with MHC incompatible donor lymph node cells together with skin isograft and donor type skin. That is, the recipient rats had either donor skin or transplanted recipient skin. Within approximately one day following transplantation, typical runt disease occurred. However, none of the donor grafts were affected, whereas all of the recipient skin displayed typical abnormalities. These data suggest that the abnormalities found in this runt's skin were caused by a specific immunological attack against it, most likely by the mononuclear cell infiltrate, and this very likely was of donor origin. Subsequently, with immunostaining and T-cell depletion (which will be discussed later), this has been firmly established. Interestingly, the changes found in the skin were not found in the oral mucosa, tongue, salivary glands, esophagus or rectum. The investigators also found that the lungs and the trachea were not affected.

From these experiments, the investigators found that one consistent feature of systemic graft-versus-host reaction is a striking enlargement of the host spleen and occasional enlargement of lymph nodes followed by involution of these organs if the mice survived. Histologically, in both spleen and lymph nodes, there is a rapid disappearance of lymphoblasts and lymphocytes from the follicular area, an abnormal proliferation of blast-like cells and no clear areas of necrosis. The thymus does not undergo enlargement, but rather rapid involution which occurs about the time of the splenomegaly or the lymphadenopathy. Histologically, there are no clear signs of cell death or destruction. The bone marrow of the mice with GVHD is pale. Although there is no clear decrease in cellularity, there is a marked decrease in erythroid cells. In the liver, the only abnormalities observed were focal areas of infiltration of the portal spaces by lymphocytes which displayed abundant mitoses. Again of interest, no abnormalities were observed in the brain, thyroid, adrenals, pancreas, salivary gland, heart, muscles, testes, ovary and adipose tissue. Moreover, the observed disease was expressed clinically and histologically in the same manner, regardless of whether spleen cells, lymph node cells, thoracic duct cells or peripheral blood leukocyte concentrates were used. Mice that developed severe GVHD developed an abnormally large liver with heavy passive congestion and yellow patches of coagulant necrosis associated with the cellular lymphoid infiltrate.

## EXPERIMENTAL GVHD

Early studies of GVHD involved no preparation of the host, and most experiments were performed simply by injecting lymph node or spleen cells from one animal into another. Under these circumstances, strains of mice differing in many minor histocompatibility loci but alike at the MHC, did not cause a graft-versus-host reaction or GVHD. Skin grafts between these mice caused prompt rejection from one normal adult donor of one strain into the other but did not cause GVHD. However, as later experiments showed, if the hosts are radiated, GVHD can be demonstrated. Even if radiation is not used, presensitization of the donor cells against the host antigens will cause GVHD.

These early experiments on GVHD also determined that the cell dosage, as well as cell type, was important. The variations in terms of total cell dose depended on the strain combination. Bone marrow was almost completely innocuous and induced tolerance of skin homograft with little risk of overt GVHD. Homogenates of the spleen, leukocyte concentrates from the peripheral blood, lymph node cells and thoracic duct cells represent grafts of increasing potency. Notably, the thymocytes were quite variable and frequently did not cause any GVHD. This clearly constituted evidence of a very different cell population found within the thymus as compared to lymph nodes. These early experiments also demonstrated that adult cells were clearly competent and caused GVHD whereas blood from fetal or neonatal donors was completely harmless due to the immaturity of those cells. The important contribution, summarized by Billingham in his Harvey lecture, was that the immunologically competent cells for graft-versus-host reaction were in fact lymphocytes.[8] Homogenized lymphocytes or lymphocytes killed by such procedures as repeated freezing/thawing or irradiation failed to cause GVHD. Moreover, the immunological competence was restricted to the small lymphocytes found either in the thoracic duct or in the peripheral blood.

Another historical observation was "parabiosis intoxication". The technique of parabiosis is the grafting of one complete animal onto the body of another. This was initially introduced by Paul Bert in 1862.[9] It had long been known that when genetically dissimilar animals were parabiotically united, vascular anastomoses became established at the lines of union. A lethal wasting syndrome known as parabiosis intoxication developed frequently where the intoxicated partner loses weight and becomes severely anemic whereas the unaffected partner gained weight and became polycythemic. The pathologic changes resembled GVHD. It was clear that the hybrid is attacked from within by immunologically competent cells-derived from the partner's blood.

The third set of experiments that helped define GVHD came from adult transplantation with what was called F1 hybrid disease. Under these combinations, offspring (F1) developed a wasting syndrome that was similar to GVHD following the inoculation of the lymphoid cells from either parental strain. These F1 hybrids are an ideal host to study GVHD since they present the inoculated cells with all the alien transplantation antigens of the other parental strain yet are genetically incapable of rejecting the grafts from either of the parental strains.

Another type of graft-versus-host reaction described was initially called "secondary disease" in radiation chimeras. This is one of the most common methods of studying GVHD today. Mice or other animals exposed to normally lethal doses of radiation recover if they are given transfusions of viable bone marrow cells from either isologous or homologous donors. These observations led to the initial clinical trials using allogeneic bone marrow for rescue following total body irradiation as a method to treat malignancies. Studies of these grafts revealed that the donor cells establish and replace the host hematopoietic cells, producing a state of chimerism. Chimerism may be complete or mixed, i.e., all donor cells as opposed to a combination of donor and residual recipient cells. When isologous donor cells are used, the majority of the mice live a normal life span and appear to be completely normal. When homologous or heterologous cells are used, survival is usually curtailed. These mice develop a disease known as secondary wasting disease and die over the course of a few months. The secondary wasting disease was felt to be the result of graft-versus-host reaction. In fact, the secondary wasting disease mimics what occurs in vivo following BMT in humans.

GVHD can also affect hematopoiesis with a reduction in host hematopoietic cells.[10] In murine models, GVHD does not have an effect on peripheral blood counts.[11] However, the hematopoietic precursors remained low. The normal peripheral blood counts were supported by increased numbers of hematopoietic progenitor cells in cycle. The clinical effects of GVHD in hematopoiesis in humans is usually not dramatic, but persistent thrombocytopenia seen in patients with GVHD may be a reflection of impaired hematopoietic stem cells.

## PREVENTION

As early as the 1960s, different methods were employed to prevent GVHD. The rationale for some of these preventive measures was as follows: if the disease that develops in the neonatal mice of one strain (strain A) injected with homologous lymphoid cells from the adult donor of a different strain (strain B) is due to graft-versus-host reaction, then concurrent injection of the infant host (strain A) with lymphoid cells from the adult host of its own strain (strain A) would confer protection against the adult's donor cells from a different strain (strain B). When such experiments were performed, mice were protected from developing GVHD. Unfortunately, this would not be feasible clinically as most patients who are offered BMT have hematological malignancies. One would not consider injecting the same cells back into the host since these would carry a high risk for potential recurrence of disease.

A second approach was the use of amethopterin, a drug which had been found to reduce the incidence of secondary disease.[12] This approach led to the use of methotrexate for the prophylaxis of GVHD following human GVHD. Another report by Cosgrove et al demonstrated that prior exposure in vitro of B6 spleen cells to a (B6 x 101) F1 liver homogenate at 10°C for about 10 hours reduced the capacity of these cells to cause secondary disease.[13] Another interesting observation, by Mathe et al, found that maintaining suspension of lymphoid or myeloid cells in Tyrode's solution or autologous serum at 37°C for an hour or two, profoundly depressed the immunologic activity.[14]

Another method for the prevention of GVHD was described in Haller. If neonatal B6 mice were splenectomized within a few hours after the intravenous injection of CBA spleen cells, the mortality from runt disease was reduced by half.[15] No protective effect was demonstrable if the spleen was removed prior to inoculation of these cells. This observation supports the hypothesis that, in intact animals, a high proportion of immunologically competent cells settle immediately in the host spleen from which a variety of anti-host responses are initiated.

It was recognized early on that because the brunt of the reaction occurs in the host lymphoid organs with lymphoid depletion in the host, the immunological competence of the host was affected. Therefore the hosts were particularly susceptible to infectious complications. Moreover, F1 hybrids injected with the parental cells failed to react against particular viruses even before the clinical onset of the disease.[16] A profound drop in immunoglobulin levels was observed in mice that developed GVHD. With the induction of tolerance in tissue homografts, several investigators found that inoculating prenatal and newborn infants with viable cells from one or more adult donors would be of use. If, later in life, the subject sustained organ damage or, for example, severe skin burns, that potential donor could be called upon for replacement purposes. In 1957, the first attempts to induce tolerance in a few newborn human babies occurred using 300 x 10⁶ parental leukocytes injected into these newborns. None of these newborns became tolerant.[17] But, in 1960, Fowler et al. reported marked prolongation of graft survival in a small group of infants transfused at birth with fresh blood for neonatal jaundice.[18] These infants were challenged with skin from the blood donors a few days later. None of these subjects appeared to suffer any harm, however, the risk of inadvertently causing GVHD discouraged further deliberate attempts to induce tolerance in newborn babies. Early in the 1960s, an attempt at therapy for immunological deficiencies such as Swiss-type agammaglobulinemia by infusion of the affected infants with adult bone marrow, suggested that GVHD in fact may have contributed to the death of these infants. A second area where GVHD occurred was the practice of intrauterine transfusion of compatible erythrocytes into the peritoneal cavity of fetuses severely affected by rhesus (Rh) antigen sensitization early in the third trimester of pregnancy. Because of the large repeated intraperitoneal transfusions, GVHD did occur.[19] Moreover, the investigators were able to establish on the basis of chromosome studies of the peripheral blood lymphocyte that chimerism was established as the cells were donated by the father.

## OTHER STUDIES

During the 1960s, various wasting syndromes in mice were described that resembled GVHD. All of these syndromes were characterized by weight loss, diarrhea, ruffled fur, abnormal gait and high mortality (Table 1.1). As early as the 1960s, with a detailed description of GVHD, the similarities between some of these wasting diseases and autoimmune diseases were noted.

### Table 1.1. Syndromes in mice resembling GVHD*

| Syndrome/disease | Cause | Susceptibility |
|---|---|---|
| Vaccine syndrome | Washed or autoclaved staphylococci or streptoccci are resistant | Newborns, germ-free animals |
| Thymectomy wasting syndrome | Removal soon after birth | Germ-free animals are resistant |
| Radiation wasting syndrome | Rescue with isologous fetal liver or bone marrow | Adults or newborns |
| Cortisol acetate wasting syndrome | Injection into newborns | Germ-free animals are more resistant |
| Virus wasting syndrome | Injection of high dose polyoma virus | Newborns |
| Antiserum wasting disease | Chronic infusion of rabbit anti-lymphocyte serum | Adults |

*All these syndromes lead to involution of the animals' lymphoid tissue (adapted from ref. 8).

The hematological abnormalities found in GVHD had been noted to be similar to systemic lupus erythematosis and related disorders in man.[20,21.] Moreover, it was found that graft-versus-host reactivity could cause or facilitate the development of malignant lymphomas. The lymphomas that occurred after transplantation were noted to be of host cell origin. These results suggested that "transplantation immunity" type mechanism may play an important role in the origin of lymphomas.

Historically, therefore, these findings led to intense research efforts into understanding the events that initiate GVHD and in assessing the clinical applicability of allogeneic bone marrow for the treatment of malignant diseases in man following total body irradiation. Data generated by these investigations have led to a continued understanding of the potential interactions which may explain the occurrence of GVHD.

### REFERENCES

1. Murphy J. The effect of adult chicken organ graft on the chicken embryo. J Exp Med 1916; 24: 1.
2. Simonsen M. Graft-versus-host reaction. Their natural history and applicability of tool of research. Prog Allergy 1962; 6: 349.
3. Simonsen M. The impact on the developing embryo and newborn animal of adult homologous cells. Acta Pathol Microbiol Scand 1957; 40: 480.
4. Billingham RE, Brent L, Medawar P. Quantitative studies on tissue transplantation immunity III. Phil Transact Roy Soc B 1953; 239: 357.

5. Billingham RE, Brent L, Medawar P. Actively acquired tolerance of grafted cells. Nature 1953; 239: 603.

6. McBride RA, Coppleson LW, Nisbet NW et al. Accelerated immunological maturation in the chick. Immunol 1966; 10: 63.

7. Gowans JL, McGregor DD, Cowen DM, Ford CE. Initiation of responses by small lymphocytes. Nature 1962; 196: 651.

8. Billingham, R. The biology of graft-versus-host reaction. Harvey Lecture 1966: 21.

9. Bert P. Experience et considerations La greffe animale. J Anat Physiol 1862: 69.

10. Iwasaki T, Fujiwara H, Shearer GM. Loss of proliferative capacity and T cell immune development potential of bone marrow from mice undergoing a graft-versus-host reaction. J Immunol 1986; 137: 3100.

11. van Dijken, P, Wimperis J, Crawford JM, Ferrara JLM. Effect of graft-versus-host disease on hematopoiesis after bone marrow transplantation in mice. Blood 1991; 78: 2773.

12. Uphoff D. Alteration of homograft reaction by a-methopterin in lethally irradiated mice treated with homologous marrow. Proc Soc Exp Biol Med 1958; 99: 651.

13. Cosgrove GE, Upton AC, Popp RA, Congdon CC. Inhibition of foreign spleen reaction by inactivation of donor cells with recipient antigens. Proc Soc Exp Biol Med 1959; 102: 525.

14. Mathe G, Amiel JL, Schwarzenberg M et al. Conditioning of immunologically competent cells by incubation at 37°C. Ann NY Acad Sci 1966; 129:355.

15. Haller J. The effect of neonatal splenectomy on mortality from runt disease in mice. Transplantation 1964; 2: 287.

16. Blaese RM, Martinez C, Good R. Immunologic incompetence of immunologically runted animals. J Exp Med 1964; 119: 211.

17. Woodruff M, Sparrow LN. Further observation on the induction of tolerance of skin homografts in rats. Transplant Bull 1957; 4: 157.

18. Fowler R, Schubert WK, West CD. Acquired partial tolerance to homologous skin grafts in the human infant at birth. Ann NY Acad Sci 1960; 87: 403.

19. Naiman JL, Punnett HH, Lischner HW et al. Possible graft-versus-host disease after intrauterine transfusion for Rh erythroblastosis fetalis. N Engl J Med 1969; 281: 697.

20. Fudenberg H, Solomon A. "Acquired agammaglobulimemia" with autoimmune hemolytic disease: graft-versus-host reaction? Vox Sanguinis 1961; 6: 68.

21. Oliner H, Schwartz R, Dameshek W. Studies in experimental autoimmune disorders. I. Clinical and laboratory features of autoimmunization (runt disease) in the mouse. Blood 1961; 17: 20.

# CHAPTER 2

# THE MAJOR HISTOCOMPATIBILITY COMPLEX (MHC)

## INTRODUCTION

Understanding GVHD or transplantation in general, as well as interactions between immune cells and the genetic control of immune responses, depends upon our knowledge of the nature of the MHC. The historical background for understanding the MHC closely parallels that of transplantation. Transplantation in chickens with different types of tissue then led Peter Gorer in the 1930s to reanalyze the field of transplantation and genetics in the mouse.[1] His work led to analysis of the blood group antigens in the few strains of inbred mice which were available at the time. He was able to identify two antigen systems. One of these antigen systems was found in all strains and differed only in quantity. This was called antigen 1 (H-1). The other antigen was found in some strains but not in others and this was called antigen 2 (H-2). Gorer and Snell demonstrated that this second antigen correlated with skin graft rejection and tumor immunity. Because these antigens were the most important in tissue rejection, they were named the major histocompatibility antigens. The genes encoding these antigens are part of the MHC. As this work evolved, it became clear that the MHC was a multigene and multiallelic complex. Gorer and Snell's work led to the demonstration that various traits were controlled by the genes of the MHC. As more and more congenic strains of mice became available (and specifically the selection of recombinant and congenic strains of mice), genetic analysis of this complex region was achieved.[2] The genes of the MHC are found in all vertebrates and consist of a number of closely linked genetic loci that function as a system. Although most of the genes identified with the MHC are involved with immune function and tissue rejection, many other genes are not. These genes are mapped to the small segment of chromosome 17 in the mouse and to the HLA (human leucocyte antigen) on the short arm of chromosome 6 in humans.

The general structure of the MHC of the mouse is comparable to those in humans, but there are many more allelic variants in humans compared to mice. Much of the H-2 complex of the mouse is divided into four main regions, the K, I, S and D regions. Boundaries of each region are defined by analyses of recombinant mice which are selected specifically for changes within the MHC complex. These congenic strains of mice which are recombinant at the MHC loci and differ at all other genetic loci have helped delineate the significance of each of these regions.

The H-2 complex is called the major histocompatibility complex because of its importance in graft rejection. The ultimate test for genetic relatedness between any two individuals has been the test for skin graft rejection of one to the other. Even the primitive protozoa, sponges, exhibit self surface recognition systems capable of identifying and destroying nonself, presumably to preserve integrity of the individuals growing in densely populated environments.[3,4] Therefore, when two genetically identical sponges (*Callyspongia diffusa*) are opposed, the individuals fuse to form a single organism. However, when two genetically dissimilar sponges are joined, there is a reaction leading to tissue destruction at the boundary between these two individuals. Self cell surface structures recognize self versus nonself and trigger effective mechanisms that lead to the destruction of the foreign tissue but not of the normal self tissue. One of the most striking features of the markers involved in the self-surface recognition phenomena is the enormous diversity or polymorphism. There are hundreds of genetically distinct sponges which have the capacity to reject one another after this type of aposition. A study of such invertebrate recognition system display three fundamental features to self/non-self recognition systems.

1.  There are self surface recognition structures.
2.  There are effective mechanisms that lead to the destruction of nonself.
3.  There is a high degree of polymorphism in the recognition structures.

These three features are important in the development of GVHD. Polymorphism is important since its high degree allows for such a self vs. non-self discrimination. The tendency has been that the more complex the organism, the higher the degree of polymorphism. Much of the genetic work done on the congenic strains has been carried out by Jan Klein and George Snell. The analyses done with these congenic strains of mice define the K and the D region of the mouse (the corresponding A, B, C regions of humans) as the so-called transplantation antigens. The recipient of the graft responds to the antigens coded by the K and D regions of the MHC. However, a major part of these reactions also seems to be coded in the I region of the mouse (the D region of humans).

The study of the genetics of the immune response in mice evolved from studying copolymers of amino acids. When a random copolymer of glutamic acid, alanine and threonine (GAT) or glutamic acid, lysine and alanine (GLA) were injected into various strains of mice, some mice made a good antibody response while others were poor responders. By selecting appropriate crosses and back-crosses, it was determined that responsiveness to each of these copolymers was probably determined by a single dominant gene. McDevitt and his co-workers demonstrated that when threonine, glutamic acid, alanine and lysine copolymer (TGAL) is emulsified with Freund's complete adjuvant and injected into a CBA or a B6 mouse, a clear difference in the amount of antibody produced by each strain was observed.[5]

CBA mice made a small amount of antibody compared to B6 mice which made a large amount of antibody. When (CBA x B6) F1 were tested, these mice made an intermediate response. Responses to these copolymers were found to map to differences in the I region of the H-2 or the MHC. As these experiments were carried further, it was discovered that the ability to be a higher responder to a given antigen was associated with the specific H-2 haplotypes. Moreover, the I region or the Ia region (for immune-associated) and the D region in man were found to be associated with the stimulation of mixed lymphocyte reaction and for graft-versus-host reaction in murine models. The strongest mixed lymphocyte reaction (MLR) were generated when the cells differed in the Ia region.

The terminology involved in the MHC may be somewhat confusing when one describes the H-2 of the mouse or the MHC of man. Class I molecules refer to the genes found in all nucleated cells. In contrast, the I region is found in the class II region and refers to the gene product of the class II region. The MHC has been found in all mammals and vertebrates studied to date. In all cases, it appears to be closely linked to class I and class II genes and associated class III genes. This linkage and the extended haplotypes found in such diverse groups of animals suggest an interesting question as to the selective constraints which have maintained this persistent linkage among these gene families.

## CLASS I REGION

The MHC spans a large chromosomal region. Within this region are the class I and class II genes. The most extensively studied and defined antigens are the class I antigens. The K and the D in the mouse or the HLA-A, HLA-B, HLA-C region of humans are referred to as class I antigens. These antigens are found in all cell types. The class I region spans approximately 2000 kb. It also contains a number of related genes termed HLA-E (on lymphoid and non-lymphoid cells), HLA-F (resting T cells and activated B cells), and HLA-G (expression limited to cytotrophoblasts) which may be functional, but these genes are not very polymorphic. Other genes such as HLA-H and HLA-J are pseudogenes. The class I antigen has been analyzed by x-ray crystallography and the structure has been elucidated.[6] The class I antigen is comprised of an α-chain polypeptide that is 45,000 daltons and is noncovalently associated with β-2 microglobulin (β2M), a 12,000 dalton polypeptide coded by a gene located in chromosome 2 in the mouse and chromosome 15 in humans. These antigens are found in virtually all nucleated cells and there is a certain homology between class I and antibody genes.

## CLASS II REGION

The I region of the mouse or the D region of man refers to class II antigens. These antigens are found more selectively in cells of the immune response system. The terminology of H-2 and class II molecules can be somewhat confusing at times. The I region of the mouse or the D region (approximately 1000 kb) in human MHC codes for the class II molecules. This MHC subregion contains genes for the class II molecules which have been characterized serologically, biochemically and have been cloned and sequenced. These molecules are composed of an α and β chain and are heterodimers. The α chains range in molecular weight from 30-33,000 and the β chains from 27-29,000 daltons. These differences are primarily due to changes in glycosylation.

Recently, the structure of the class II molecule has been elucidated by x-ray crystallography. From similarities in the primary structure of class I and class II MHC molecules, a proposed model for a class II MHC binding site appears to have been corroborated by recent data suggesting that this model is consistent with the observed three dimensional structure of the class II molecule.[7,8] It appears that the structure of the MHC class II molecule is remarkably similar to the structure of the class I molecule. However, there are some significant differences between these two molecules. The class I peptide-binding pocket appears to be blocked at either end and thus imposes severe restrictions on the size of peptides it can accommodate. These peptides are approximately 8-10 residues. The longer peptides bulge out in the middle.[9] The class II molecules, however, allow peptides to protrude from the groove and consequently longer peptides can be accommodated. The average number of amino acids appears to be 15-18 residues and therefore there is no need for bulging at the middle.[10] Studies of self peptide eluded from purified class II molecules have established the size heterogeneity. These peptides are thought to bind through a central core of conserved amino acid with "ragged" ends. With this model, promiscuous peptides capable of binding to many different MHC class II molecules have been identified.[10,11] There is no obvious parallel for this with class I molecules. It is interesting to speculate that the binding of the peptide to MHC class II molecules may be governed by different rules than those of the class I molecule. This differential binding may be related to the ability to elicit GVHD.

The major surprise is that the DR1 molecule which has been analyzed crystallographically is a heterodimer; that is, the one MHC molecule is a dimer. It appears that these class II MHC molecules come in pairs of dimers. It is as if this pair of dimers may allow for simultaneous interaction with two T-cell receptor complexes. Alternatively, in antigen-presenting cells, this dimerization may induce expression of costimulatory molecules. It is very interesting to speculate whether low affinity in the dimer interaction may be an important feature in T-cell activation, i.e., potentially a mechanism for a critical mass of high affinity binding peptides to be present in the MHC class II pocket before the T cell is activated. Unless a specific mechanism exists for the simultaneous presence of the same peptide in both grooves, the normal state of these dimers would be to contain two different peptides, only one specific for any given T cell. This may not be sufficient for T-cell activation.

These class II molecules serve as restricting elements that permit regulatory T cells to view antigen in the context of self or the surface of other T cells, macrophages, B cells or antigen-presenting cells.[7] These class II genes and their products appear to control the proliferation of regulatory T-cells, as well as the effector function carried out by these T cells, such as amplification of T-cell subsets and B-cell proliferation. There are several structural similarities between class I, class II molecules and β-2 microglobulin and antibodies. It is the interaction between the class II molecule, antigen and the T-cell receptor that is the critical event in the initiation of an

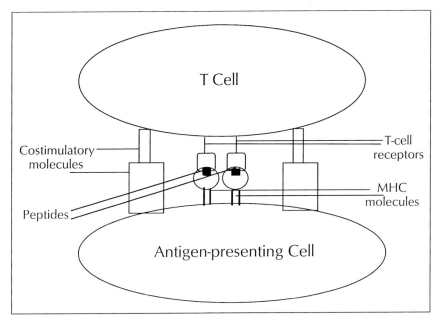

*Fig. 2.1. Schematic model of the trimolecular interaction in antigen presentation involving the T-cell receptor, antigen-presenting cell and the peptide. Costimulatory molecules are also an important part in determining the T-cell response.*

immune response (Fig. 2.1). The data on the amino acid sequence and polymorphism for the MHC class II molecules, combined with the specific structural information on the T-cell receptor and the antigen itself, may allow detailed understanding of the interactions that are required for the immune response to occur. Most of the genes of the MHC are highly polymorphic with many allelic forms. Alloreactivity is one of the results when T cells from one individual recognizes allelic differences in non-self MHC antigens. One of the results of this alloreactivity is GVHD.

The most centromeric region of the HLA is the class II region. In humans this region codes for the HLA-DR, HLA-DQ and HLA-DP. This region also includes the genes involved in antigen processing such as the proteosome-related genes encoding the low molecular weight proteins (LMP) and the genes encoding the peptide transporters, the so called ABC (ATP-binding cassette) transporters. The stretch of DNA, however, could possibly encode for more than 50 separate genes. Several genes found in this region have no obvious association with the immune system. Two such genes are the collagen gene type 11A2 and RING 3 gene homologous to the Drosophila female sterile homeotic.

There are three subregions which have also been well identified, the DR, DQ and DP. Two other regions, DO and DZ, have also been studied. Each of these regions contain several beta chains and at least one α chain. The DR subregion has been the most studied. It contains at least one α chain and three β chains. The HLA-DQ region contains five genes, two α and three β genes. Only the α1 and β1 gene products are known to be expressed. The HLA-DP region contains four genes, two α and two β genes. Only the α1 and β1 gene products are known to be expressed. The class II region contains additional genes such as the α chain-like genes DMA and DNA, and the β chain-like genes DMB and DOB. The function of these genes is presently unknown.

## CLASS III REGION

Class III genes are located between the class I and II regions. This area spans approximately 700 kb and at least 36 genes have been located in this area. Several of these genes encode for proteins that are important in immune functions such as some of the complement cascade factors (C2, C4, Bf), two genes encoding for tumor necrosis factor (TNF α and β), and two heat shock proteins (Hsp 70 and 1H.C4). The other proteins are not known to be associated with the immune system. For example, the steroid hormone biosynthesis enzyme 21-hydroxylase is found in this region. The function of many of the genes in this region remains unknown.

## ABERRANT MHC EXPRESSION

Aberrant MHC antigen expression of class I or class II antigens may also be important in the pathophysiology of acute GVHD.[12] Using a rat model, Parfrey et al demonstrated that an early lymphoproliferative phase coincided with MHC antigen induction on epithelial cells in several tissues. Following this antigen induction, there is a mononuclear cell infiltration and cell injury at these particular sites. The nonlymphoid tissue injury is confined to epithelial cells that aberrantly express MHC antigens. Moreover, acute GVHD was found to be associated with a striking increase in the number of MHC class II-positive interstitial dendritic cells (predominantly of host origin) in both target and non-target cells. This correlation suggests that these MHC class II antigens are involved in the selection of tissue for destruction in GVHD. Furthermore, class II antigens may be more important than class I antigens in determining cell injury. This observation is consistent with the observation that class II disparity is associated with stronger GVHD compared to class I differences.[13,14] Expression of class II antigens was clearly not the only factor associated with GVHD since various other organs expressed aberrant class II antigens and did not result in GVHD. These authors speculate whether allogeneic T cells have a higher affinity for class II antigens when these antigens are complexed to epithelial cell antigens.

## REFERENCES

1. Gorer P. The detection of antigenic differences in mouse erythrocytes by development of immune sera. Br Med Bull 1936; 17: 50.
2. Klein J. The Natural History of the Major Histocompatibility Complex. New York: Wiley and Sons 1986.
3. Hildeman WH, Jokiel PJ, Bigger CH, Johnston IS. Allogeneic polymorphism and alloimmune memory in the coral, *Montispora verrucosa*. Transplantation 1980; 30: 297.
4. Hildeman WH, Johnson IS, Jokiel PL. Immune complex in the lowest metazoan phyllum: Transplantation immunity in sponges. Science 1979; 204: 420.
5. McDevitt HO, Chinitz A. Genetic control of the antibody response: Relationship between immune response and histocompatibility (H-2) type. Science 1969; 163: 1207.

6. Bjorkman PJ, Saper M, Samraoui B et al. Structure of human class I histo-compatibility antigen, HLA-A2. Nature 1987; 329: 506.

7. Brown JH, Jardetsky T, Saper MA et al. A hypothetical model of the foreign antigen binding site of class II histocompatibility molecules. Nature 1988; 337: 845.

8. Brown JH, Jardetsky T, Gorga JC et al. Three-dimensional structure of the human class II histocompatibility antigen HLA-DR1. Nature 1993; 364: 33.

9. Guo H-C, Jardetzky TS, Garrett TP et al. Different length peptides bind to HLA-Aw68 similarly at their ends but bulge out in the middle. Nature 1992; 360: 36.

10. Chicz RM, Urban RG, Gorga JC et al. Specificity and promiscuity among naturally processed peptides bound to HLA-DR alleles. J Exp Med 1993; 178: 27.

11. Sinigaglia F, Guttinger M, Kilgus J et al. A malaria T-cell epitope recognition in association with most mouse and human MHC class II molecules. Nature 1988; 336: 778.

12. Parfrey NA, Ste-Croix H, Prud'homme GJ. Evidence that nonlymphoid tissue injury in acute graft-versus-host disease is limited to epithelial cells aberrantly expressing MHC antigens. Transplantation 1989; 48: 655.

13. Hamilton BL, Parkman R. Kinetics of the anti-recipient cytotoxic cell response of mice with minor antigen graft-vs-host disease. J Immunol 1982; 128:376.

14. Klein J, Pack JM. Graft-versus-host reaction across different regions of the H-2 complex of the mouse. J Exp Med 1973; 137: 1213.

# CHAPTER 3

# ETIOLOGY OF GRAFT-VERSUS-HOST DISEASE

## INTRODUCTION

GVHD is a major barrier to effective bone marrow transplantation in humans. The incidence of GVHD varies from 9-76% (average 30%) even though recipient and donor sibling pairs are matched at the HLA loci (A,B,DR) and intensive immunosuppression is used.[1-4] The mortality rate can be as high as 50% in patients who develop GVHD. GVHD can result when immunocompetent allogeneic cells encounter foreign cells after transplantation. This is similar to the recognition process that occurs after organ transplantation and graft rejection. Earlier experiments demonstrated that cells which are not matched at the MHC cause this allogeneic reaction and GVHD.

## WHY DOES GVHD OCCUR?

What is the specificity of GVHD when donor and recipient are HLA identical? There is extensive literature in various experimental animal models as to the specific cellular requirements for GVHD (Table 3.1). The most widely utilized experimental animals for GVHD studies are murine models. Studies of GVHD show differences in the MHC class I, class II or minor histocompatibility antigen result in varying outcomes. The subpopulations of T cells (CD4+, CD8+ or both) that initiate GVHD in response to the MHC or minor histocompatibility antigens vary with specific donor/recipient combinations tested.[5,6] Data demonstrate that 10 times fewer cells were necessary to establish GVHD in congenic strains differing in the class II region compared to differences in the class I region.[7] Moreover, GVHD in man is more prominent when the donor/recipient pairs are mismatched in the DR region. The major focus will be on disparities in minor histocompatibility antigens which reflect what occurs in human bone marrow transplantation where GVHD

---

**Table 3.1 Cells implicated in GVHD**

Helper T cells
Alloreactive cytotoxic T cells
Natural killer (NK) cells
Natural killer-like cells
Lymphokine-activated killer (LAK) cells

---

remains a problem even though donor/recipients are matched at the MHC loci. Occasionally the results observed from such experimental models are noncomplementary and even directly contradictory. The differences in murine models, i.e., major or minor histocompatibility differences, appear to dictate which type of effector cells are important. For example, when mice are incompatible in certain minor histocompatibility antigens, lethal graft-versus-host response of these T cells involves a recognition of a limited number of those minor antigens. There is a pattern of immunodominant antigen recognition in GVHD. Death only occurs with large doses of allogeneic T cells and the overall mortality is also related to the cleanliness of the mouse colony.

But what causes GVHD when donor/recipients are matched at the MHC? Under these circumstances, GVHD results from the recognition of recipient histocompatibility antigens ("minor" histocompatibility antigens) by the contaminating T cells in the donor marrow. Although these antigens are called minor histocompatibility antigens, to differentiate them from the MHC, many of these antigens are far from being of "minor" significance clinically. Experimental models during the 1960-70s implicated lymphocytes, specifically T cells, in the development of GVHD.[8] Similar effects are seen in patients after allogeneic BMT. Experiments with heterologous antithymocyte globulin, and more recently with specific T-cell subset depletion, have unequivocally demonstrated that donor T cells are a prerequisite for GVHD.[9-12] Unfortunately, T-cell depletion in humans prevents GVHD, but is associated with increased graft failure and relapse with no improvement in overall survival.[13]

## T-CELL INVOLVEMENT

Investigators have shown that removing T cells from donor marrow prevents acute GVHD. Much of the early data were obtained from murine models. Destruction of donor reactive T cells of host origin, followed by intrathymic clonal deletion of these cells, was suggested as one possible mechanism in preventing GVHD in cyclophosphamide-induced tolerant mice.[14] Several clinical studies confirmed the decreased incidence of acute GVHD; however, various associated problems such as increased graft failure and leukemic relapse also result after T-cell depletion. Many attempts have been made to define the cellular subsets and mechanisms required for engraftment and graft-versus-leukemia effect and alternative approaches for T-cell depletion continue to be explored. Clinical studies suggest that T cells from the donor help to eliminate, remove or inactivate residual host lymphocytes which have survived the conditioning regimen and therefore are able to cause graft rejection.[15] Donor T cells also contribute to lung damage from total body irradiation.[16] The addition of T cells to marrow in this murine model did not aid engraftment but significantly increased pulmonary toxicity.

Investigators from the Institute Gustave Roussy analyzed the T-cell receptor variability in transplanted patients with acute GVHD. When the first signs of engraftment were detectable and at the time of GVHD diagnosis, the αβ T-cell receptor was studied. The Vα and Vβ gene usage were analyzed after cDNA amplification by the polymerase chain reaction (PCR) of the peripheral blood mononuclear cells and skin samples from three patients with grade II cutaneous GVHD. All the Vα and Vβ subfamilies were represented in the peripheral blood RNA. Lymphocytes infiltrating the GVHD skin also expressed a large series of Vα and Vβ subfamily specificities. Interestingly, however, the Vα and Vβ differed between the peripheral blood and the skin. Unfortunately it is not known whether the lymphocytes derived from actual T-cell precursors simply reflect the expansion of mature T lymphocytes present in the graft.[17]

## T-CELL PRECURSORS

It is unclear if the immunodominance for the occurrence of GVHD due to minor histocompatibility differences corresponds with the ability to generate cytotoxic T lymphocytes in vitro.[18,19] Some cytotoxic T-cell immunity against minor histocompatibility antigens is assumed to contribute to the development of GVHD in recipients of HLA identical bone marrow, yet there is no clear correlation between the presence of the cytotoxic T cells and the occurrence of GVHD. In one study, 16 patients were studied between 1 and 25 months after grafting.[18] Four of five patients who developed acute GVHD and five of five patients with chronic GVHD had demonstrable specific anti-host cytotoxic T-cell activity. However, in five of six patients with no clinical signs of GVHD, anti-host cytotoxic T cells were also detected. The anti-host T-cell activity appeared within the first three months, increased to maximum activity between three and six months and then disappeared. These results suggest that patients with chronic GVHD develop higher and more persistent levels of anti-host cytotoxic T-cell activity compared to those who do not have GVHD. A second study on the mechanism of GVHD at the level of cytotoxic T-cell precursors indicated that the expansion of minor histocompatibility-specific CTL precursors was related to the clinical manifestation of severe GVHD.[20] There was a severe depletion of alloreactive CTL precursors following BMT. However, determination of minor histocompatibility-specific CTL precursors did not predict the occurrence of GVHD.

A recent study partly corroborates these observations and was able to correlate the occurrence of GVHD with minor histocompatibility antigen-specific cytotoxic T cells.[21] Host-specific cytotoxic T cells were detected exclusively in the peripheral blood of patients with acute GVHD after BMT between HLA-matched sibling pairs. The target antigens from these host-specific CTLs were simultaneously expressed on several host-cell lines. This study suggested that "extensive" GVHD is accompanied by marked increase in the minor histocompatibility antigen-specific cytotoxic T-cell precursor and that this selection allows for the cloning of specific T-cell clones. By using a different approach of limiting dilution analysis of host reactive cytotoxic donor T cells, other investigators have been successful in predicting the incidence and severity of acute GVHD following grafting between phenotypically HLA-matched unrelated donors.[22,23] Limiting dilution assay of cytotoxic T-cell precursor frequencies in patients with clinical GVHD were compared to those who did not develop GVHD. There was a significant correlation between high CTL precursor frequencies prior to BMT and the severity of acute GVHD after HLA, A, B, DR matched and unrelated donor transplants using T-cell depleted marrow. Such an assay may be useful for the selection of a matched unrelated donor. It is possible, however, that with more specific tissue typing such as PCR analysis, this high frequency of CTL precursors would diminish significantly. Matching for histocompatibility antigens in matched unrelated donors has relied on serological HLA, A, B, C, DR and DQ typing along with a negative reaction to mixed lymphocyte cultures. Most recently, PCR typing for DR antigens has also been instituted. Since typing for HLA DP is not routine, differences for these molecules would only be detected indirectly if they induce a significant proliferation in the primary MLR response. However, this is not always the case. One study has suggested that DP differences may account for a high incidence of acute GVHD in matched unrelated donors.[24] This cytotoxic T lymphocyte precursor frequency shows better correlation with a degree of incompatibility defined by serotyping than the mixed lymphocyte cultures. This assay, however, was not predictive for GVHD in HLA-matched sibling pairs. De Bueger et al attempted to define the effector mechanisms inducing the cutaneous lesions observed in GVHD. They questioned if infiltrating CD8+ T cells could account for cutaneous GVHD.[25] These investigators tested whether host minor histocompatibility antigen-reactive cytotoxic T cells could directly lyse the epidermal cell layer. The results suggested that some cytotoxic T cells do have the in vitro potential to destroy these epidermal cells whereas others do not. This restriction in terms of the response may be linked to the tissue distribution where the minor histocompatibility antigens are expressed.

Another study assessed the frequency with which host-specific interleukin-2 (IL-2) secreting donor T-cell precursors occurred prior to undergoing BMT. The results demonstrate that the frequency of such cells correlates with the development of acute GVHD in HLA-matched recipients.[26] The involvement of such lymphokine secreting cells is corroborated by the detection of host-specific noncytolytic T cells rather than cytolytic T cells after BMT and correlates with the incidence and severity of GVHD.[18,27] The data suggest that the donor-responding capacity is predictive of the development of GVHD. By modifying the mixed lymphocyte culture, alloreactivity can be measured by the mixed lymphocyte culture and normalized by the pool response (third-party cells).[28,29] This phenomena reflects donor T-cell proliferation induced by the pool of alloreactive presenting cells (from randomly selected individuals), although not specificity for host antigens. Overall, these findings demonstrate that cytotoxic T cells have an effector role in GVHD, but other cells and risk factors are also involved. The several experiments described above suggest that CTLs are an important effector cell in GVHD; however, the identification of host-specific CTLs is not helpful in predicting GVHD across minor histocompatibility antigens, but appears to be useful in MHC mismatched unrelated donor bone marrow transplantation.

Another attempt to prevent lethal GVHD uses ex vivo treatment of murine splenocyte-supplemented bone marrow innocula with mafosfamide prior to allogeneic transplantation.[30] Mice receiving placebo-treated splenocytes supplemented bone marrow are likely to develop symptoms of severe GVHD. Treatment of the donor cells with 160 mM mafosfamide for 30 minutes results in a marked increase in animal survival without GVHD. A four-fold higher dose of mafosfamide results in improved survival. However, at this higher dose, host resistance to engraftment occurs as indicated by the low percentage of donor mononuclear cells in the peripheral blood of the survivors. Treatment of the donor cells with a four-fold lower dose of mafosfamide results in a slight increase in survival; however, all the animals develop symptoms of GVHD. These data suggest that mafosfamide as well as monoclonal antibodies and immunotoxin may be used in depleting T cells. The data also suggest that GVHD-causing T lymphocytes are more sensitive to mafosfamide than are hematopoietic-repopulating cells. This is consistent with the observation that phytohemagglutinin- and Concanavalin A- stimulated T lymphocyte proliferation is more sensitive to inhibition by mafosfamide than is the proliferation of murine pluripotent hematopoietic stem cells. The difference in the sensitivity may be related to the ability of each cell population to detoxify the drug.

One interesting subgroup is the transplantation of fetal liver cells to treat severe immunodeficiencies, hematological disorders and inborn errors of metabolism.[31] This treatment is successful in approximately two-thirds of the patients evaluable when there is not a matched donor for bone marrow transplantation. Surprisingly, the analysis of T lymphocytes from the transplanted patients demonstrates that they are derived from the donor HLA-mismatched stem cells. Despite this major incompatibility, tolerance of these cells is stable and GVHD is limited. Antigen presentation between donor-derived T cells and host-derived antigen-presenting cells occurs. The immature T or fetal cells from the donor may explain the lack of GVHD. The immaturity of the fetal recipients subjected to the in utero fetal liver transplant explains a lack of rejection.

## T-CELL PHENOTYPES

Many investigators have tried to describe which T-cell phenotype is responsible for GVHD. Experimental evidence for the involvement of CD4[+] and CD8[+] T-cell subsets in GVHD has been reviewed.[32] Specifically, for mice identical at the MHC but mismatched at multiple minor histocompatibility antigens, depletion of CD8[+] T cells is sufficient to reduce and prevent GVHD in some donor/host combinations. In certain models, CD8[+] T cells play an important role in the development of disease directed at these minor histocompatibility antigens. There are some indications that highly purified populations of these cells are capable of mediating GVHD without apparent help from mature donor-derived CD4[+] T cells. CD4[+] T cells in the innoculum enhances the potential to cause GVHD of these CD8[+] cells. This enhancement is observed at both low and high doses of CD4[+] cells. CD4[+] T cells have also been observed to cause GVHD across minor histocompatibility antigen differences in certain strain combinations without additional CD8[+] T cells. Therefore, the current results indicate that CD4[+] cells are capable of mediating acute GVHD in certain strain combinations.[33] However, CD4[+] cells can also protect in anti-MHC class II GVHD.[34] In this murine model of GVHD, low doses of CD4[+] cells, when combined with donor bone marrow, resulted in acute lethal GVHD. But large doses of CD4[+] cells administered with bone marrow paradoxically resulted in only limited mortality, and most of the recipients had no ill effects. The author suggests that large doses of CD4[+]cells enable the host to repel pathogens, especially in the gut, and therefore GVHD becomes sublethal.

It is clear that CD8[+] cells which mediate GVHD across minor histocompatibility barriers are similar to those which mediate anti-class I GVHD across major histocompatibility barriers. These CD8[+] cells appear to function independently from CD4[+] cells which commonly provide help in the form of IL-2.[34] CD8[+] cells found after the occurrence of GVHD may be driven by endogenous production of IL-2. CD8[+] cells responding to this graft-versus-host reaction can produce other lymphokines, such as IL-3, upon further activation with an anti-CD3 antibody.[35] It is unclear whether these are a unique population of CD8[+] cells or if all CD8[+] cells have some possibility for limited IL-2 production. One interesting possibility is that these helper-independent CD8[+] cells may have to express an IL-1 receptor in order to become activated and produce IL-2.[36,37] These data led to a comparison of the occurrence of GVHD from purified T cells in six donors/host pairs.[38] The results demonstrated that the CD8[+] T cells were effective mediators of GVHD in all six whereas CD4[+] cells induced GVHD in only two of these combinations. These data suggest that immunogenetic factors related to the MHC subtype may be responsible for the relative importance of each T-cell subset in the occurrence of GVHD. Endogenous factors, such as other potential cytokines or endogenous factors such as microbial infection or other environmental antigens presented in association with MHC class II molecules in vivo, may be involved in the activation of CD4[+] T cells in addition to non-MHC-encoded immunogenic determinants in mice. One such example in mice is the Mls system.[39]

Different transplantation models across minor histocompatibility barriers suggest that CD4[+] T cells are important. Ex vivo depletion of CD4[+] T cells eliminated graft-versus-host associated mortality in a B10.BR donor mouse transplanted into AKR recipient murine model.[40] Removal of CD8[+] T cells in the murine model did not effect overall survival. However, even in this murine model, CD8[+] cytotoxic T lymphocytes from B10 BR mice are capable of causing lethal GVHD in AKR mice in the absence of T helper cells. This suggests that both T-cell subsets can mediate GVHD reactivity in minor histocompatibility antigens. One suggestion is that CD8[+] cytotoxic T cells may operate independently of any helper input; however, the presence of CD4[+] helper cells can accelerate the response.[41] CD4[+] cells clearly play an important part in GVHD occurring across minor histocompatibility barriers. This has been shown to be important even in humans.[42]

Further evidence that T cells are important in the occurrence of GVHD comes from in vivo use of monoclonal antibodies directed against T cells. In one study, unmodified IgG$_{2b}$ anti-T-cell monoclonal antibody effectively reduced GVHD when given after bone marrow reconstitution. Allogeneic spleen cells were injected into the host followed by use of monoclonal antibody directed against either helper or cytotoxic T cells.[43] Results indicated that intravenous or intraperitoneal administration of an anti-T-cell monoclonal antibody, Thy-1 (a pan T-cell marker), prevented GVHD across a major histocompatibility barrier. In this murine model, purified CD4[+] cells were able to induce lethal GVHD where the CD8[+] T cells were not. These results argue for a dominant role of the CD4[+] T-cell subset. However, when monoclonal antibodies were directed against either CD4[+] or CD8[+] cells, both resulted in a substantial decrease in the mortality rate. Since CD8[+] T cells in this strain combination are not able to induce lethal

GVHD alone, they might depend on the help of CD4+ T cells or their product.[43] Thus, as discussed earlier, the relative roles of CD4+ and CD8+ T cells remain controversial. It seems that with class I incompatibility, CD8+ T cells are essential whereas, with class II MHC incompatibilities, CD4+ T cells are important. CD4+ cells played a predominant role in GVHD in most experimental models with both MHC and non-MHC incompatibilities. In alloimmune responses, synergy between CD4+ and CD8+ cells has been shown in vivo for the mediation of graft rejection, as well as in vitro for generation of cytotoxic T cells.[44,45] It is unclear whether true synergy between CD4+ and CD8+ cells occurs in GVHD. Another study in rats confirmed the differences in alloreactivity between the strains tested and suggested that the differences may be due to alternate requirements for alloactivation of T-cell subsets. In rats with a high responder subset of T cells to alloantigens, either subset may be sufficient to induce lethal GVHD. In contrast, low responder strains appear to require a mixture of both CD4+ and CD8+ cells to induce lethal GVHD.[46]

GVHD has been studied through immunization of F1 hybrid host with low doses of parental cells. This model demonstrates that the F1 hybrid responds through the receptor of the unshared MHC antigen on the immunizing cells, inducing a specific resistance to a GVHD challenge from the cells of the same parental strain. This graft-versus-host resistance may be induced by tolerant cell populations. Preliminary data suggest that the intensity of GVHD response can be moderated by prior injection of small numbers of cells of the relevant parental strain and indicates that parental cells do not express antigens recognized by the F1 hybrid. The cellular mechanism(s) of transplantation tolerance are not fully understood. Both clonal deletion and specific suppression have been proposed as possible mechanisms.[47,48] These data suggest that suppression in tolerant animals occurs by the generation of clones of alloinsensitive cells. This is supported by the finding that tolerant animals have very low levels of specific cytotoxic T-cell precursors.[49] However, there are cell populations from tolerant animals that appear to have the capacity to induce F1 hybrid resistance to GVHD responses, which would suggest that these cells are not clonally deleted.

A portion of T lymphocytes bearing the γδ and the αβ T-cell antigen receptors were studied in histological sections of skin of normal subjects and of patients suffering from acute GVHD. The proportion of γδ T cells overall was low but significantly higher in the skin of patients with GVHD than those without GVHD. These results suggested that these cells could play an important role in GVHD.[50] However, further studies investigating the distribution of these γδ T cells in the liver, intestine and major lymphoid organs after bone marrow transplantation showed that the number of γδ T cells is in proportion to the total number of CD3+ cells and did not differ from that found in normal tissue. This would suggest that there is no clear evidence that γδ T cells play a particularly important role in T-cell regeneration after marrow transplantation or that they are associated with the pathophysiology of acute GVHD.[51]

Although there is no doubt that T cells are important in GHVD, there is still no consensus on the precise contribution of T-cell subsets in the induction of acute GVHD. An example of this is that graft-versus-host reactions have been observed after transfer of spleen cells from nude mice. These mice are athymic and are thought not to contain mature T lymphocytes, yet transfer of bone marrow cells of these animals elicit significant graft-versus-host reactions.[52,53] However, it is now known that IL-2 induces the presence of T cells in nude mice. This mechanism may cause the graft-versus-host reaction.

Progress in some of these studies, however, needs to be assessed in light of the current understanding of T-cell and cytokine responses. When donor recipient cells are selected for in a positive sense, i.e., by "panning", such techniques would not regularly detect any CD4[+] influence based solely on cytokine production. In contrast, negative selection with depletion using a monoclonal antibody and complement to delete a specific T-cell subset may more rarely detect the influence of a cytokine producer. Negative selection may more likely detect the presence of other effectors in the system. Thus, for example, one group has used an anti-Thy1 monoclonal antibody to deplete mature and immature T cells. Using this antibody, the possibility exists that between one quarter and one third of the observed GVHD may be due to T cells not displaying either the CD4[+] or CD8[+] differentiating antigen at the time of transplant.[41] Data supports the observation that there may be at least two effector cell components to GVHD across minor histocompatibility barriers. One component is the mature CTLs already present among the donor cells at the time of transplant. The other is an immature donor type CTL precursor which, following transplantation, may differentiate into a mature anti-recipient CTL.[6,54] A second line of evidence comes from studies in humans where an in vitro assay to predict GVHD was developed in matched unrelated donor transplants. A significant correlation between the frequency of donor CTL precursors present prior to transplant and the resultant severity of GVHD in the matched unrelated transplants was demonstrated.[41] These results were even predictive when the donor cells were depleted for differentiated T cells using anti-CD7 and anti-CD8 monoclonal antibody and complement before transplantation.[23] The data suggest that undifferentiated cytotoxic T-cell precursors may influence the development of GVHD.

In summary, T cells are important in the development of GVHD. The different models reviewed here suggest that CD4[+], CD8[+] or both are important in the occurrence of GVHD. Many of the discrepancies that exist are likely due to the unique animal models used. Therefore, the animal models do not provide a cohesive schema for the cellular requirements for GVHD. However, given the unique requirements of CD4[+] cells in most cellular immune responses, one possible mechanism is that CD4[+] cells are the critical cells in the afferent arm for the induction of GVHD and CD8[+] cells are part of the efferent arm in GVHD.

Other data, however, demonstrate that enhancement of engraftment by T cells in T-cell depleted bone marrow allograft is mediated by CD8[+] cells and not by CD4[+] T cells.[55] Moreover, it appears that the CD8[+] cells which enhanced engraftment are devoid of GVHD activity. In other allogeneic BMT data in vivo administration of anti-Lyt 2.2 monoclonal antibody and anti-CD4 monoclonal antibody into recipient mice, implicated that the effector cells of lethal GVHD were predominantly CD4[+] cells. However, for the induction of sub acute lethal GVHD, the combination of both

CD8[+] and CD4[+] cells were necessary. The effector mechanism appears, therefore, to vary in different strain combinations although the donor/recipient histoincompatibility is the same.[56] These models involved B6 cells transferred into the irradiated Balb-c nu/nu compared to B6 transferred into Balb/c CB6F1 nu/nu.

## NATURAL KILLER AND NATURAL KILLER-LIKE CELLS

While alloreactive T cells are the primary mediators of GVHD, there are other cells which may act as effectors of GVHD. For example, there is evidence to suggest that natural killer (NK) cells may also be important in acute GVHD. Augmented NK activity is observed in the peripheral blood of patients who develop acute GVHD.[57] NK cells are also found in the tissues of mice, rats and human bone marrow recipients during GVHD.[58-60] The characteristic mononuclear cells infiltrating the target organs of mice with acute GVHD following MHC identical donor BMT also demonstrate large granular lymphocytes.[61] These cells are often found in close proximity to dying or dead epithelial cells in the skin, liver and colon. Analysis of the phenotype of these putative effectors show these cells to be $Thy1^+$, $ASGM_1^+$, $Mac1^+$, $Lyt-1^-$, $Lyt2^-$, $Ia^-$, which is characteristic of large granular lymphocytes. The cytolytic function in GVHD splenocytes indicates high natural killer activity and low cytolytic T-cell activity. The most compelling evidence for the involvement of NK cells in GVHD comes from murine models in which the effect of NK cells has been removed, either by antibody and complement depletion or by the use of mice that are congenitally NK cell-deficient. GVHD can be prevented by treating recipient mice with anti-asialo $GM_1$ ganglioside antibody.[62,63] A number of investigators have used animal models to study the role of NK cells in GVHD and determine whether these effector cells are of donor or host origin. Some have found that in-vivo treatment of recipient but not donor mice with anti-asialo $GM_1$ antibody reduced GVHD mortality. This led to the conclusion that NK cells of the host are the effector cells of GVHD. Ghayur et al identified an inducible anti-asialo $GM_1$ population.[64] Therefore, anti-asialo $GM_1$ treatment may eliminate NK cells of the donor, as well as that of the host.

These observations are even more complex since studies suggest that, in acute GVHD, there are several "NK-like" cells with a lytic repertoire that includes target cells resistant to lysis by conventional NK targets.[65] These NK-like cells are asialo $GM_1^+$, $Thy1^+$, $Lyt2^-$, $L3T4^-$ and are of donor origin.[66] These NK-like cells are dependent on type 1 interferon. When a monoclonal antibody, NK1.1 (which recognizes an allotypic determinant on NK cells of $H-2^b$ mice) is used for depletion of these cells from the graft, lethal GVHD was prevented. But this prevention occurred only if the donor had been injected with an interferon inducer.[67] Moreover, although wasting and mortality are prevented, these mice still developed splenomegaly and immunosuppression, two hallmarks of the GVHD.[67,68] These data support the conclusion that lethal GVHD may occur from contribution in part by these NK or NK-like cells. Selective NK depletion did not impair the engraftment process and resulted in less GHVD. However, NK1.1-depleted donor graft recipients had a significantly increased mortality, suggesting that the NK depletion may reduce immune protective function with an increased risk of infection post-transplantation.[68]

These observations about NK and NK-like cells have taken a new twist. Although originally described as an NK-specific marker, NK1.1 was recently shown to be co-expressed with CD3 and the T-cell receptor (TCR) $\alpha/\beta$ in a small population of CD4$^-$/CD8$^-$ lymphocytes.[69,70] It is possible that the effector cells removed by this monoclonal antibody are a population of T cells. Thus, the effect of anti-asialo GM$_1$ could be due to depletion of cells other than NK cells. These other cells do not appear to be mature T cells. Studies using this monoclonal antibody in murine models showed that depletion of these NK and NK-like cells do not result in lack of engraftment (an important adverse effect of T-cell depletion) and there is no loss of graft-versus-leukemia reactivity.[68,71] There is an associated decrease in the incidence of moderate to severe GVHD. Since depletion of CD4$^+$ T cells completely eliminates GVHD reactivity in the B10.BR/AKR murine model, NK cells appear to play a role as secondary GVH effector cells in response to T-cell activation.[40] CD8$^+$ depletion also significantly reduces GVHD-induced mortality compared with a non-T-cell depleted group.[71] These results are in agreement with a two phase model of GVHD has been proposed where T cells secrete lymphokine and activate NK cells as co-effector cells.[72]

A second approach in using asialo GM$_1$ antibody attempted to enrich cells which may protect against GVHD. These data contradict that presented above. Following total lymphoid irradiation (TLI), non-T-cell-depleted allogeneic bone marrow can be given with stable chimerism without GVHD occurring.[73] After TLI, there is an expansion of natural suppressor (NS) cells in the spleen which correlated with the absence of GVHD.[74] Fresh NS cells belong to the null cell lineage, i.e., non-T, non-B, non-macrophage, Sca1$^-$. Cloned NS cells are asialo GM$_1$$^+$.[75] Injecting anti-asialo GM$_1$ antibodies into mice that received TLI increases the incidence of GVHD. Depletion of asialo GM$_1$$^+$ cells from donor bone marrow also facilitates the occurrence of GVHD.[74,76]

The last model for the protective role of a subset of asialo GM$_1$ cells comes from removing asialo GM$_1$$^+$ cells from syngeneic bone marrow. This is followed by BMT, in which T-cell depleted syngeneic and allogeneic bone marrow cells are administered to a lethally irradiated mouse. In this model, lethal GVHD only occurs in the group of mice receiving syngeneic bone marrow from which asialo GM$_1$$^+$ cells were depleted prior to infusion. Therefore, asialo GM$_1$ cells from both recipient, as well as the donor origin, can suppress the occurrence of GVHD.

Asialo GM$_1$ antigen is expressed on several cell types such as cultured natural suppressor cells, natural killer cells, lymphokine-activated killer (LAK) cells, activated cytotoxic T cells, as well as macrophages.[77-81] Thus, these data appear to be contradictory in nature, where removal of asialo GM$_1$ cells may result in protection or enhancement of GVHD. These variations may be related to differences in how these experiments were performed. Differences in minor versus major histocompatibility antigens may partially explain some of these results; use of spleen cell versus bone marrow again may partially explain others. Finally, TBI versus TLI may skew results towards protection rather than GVHD via expansion of NS cells. It is clear, however, that we do not yet fully understand the contribution of these cells in GVHD.

Evaluation of long-term serial changes in the immunologic state following allogeneic BMT has also been performed.[82] The absolute number of CD2, CD20 and DR+ cells recovered their normal range in three months, one year and two years, respectively, after BMT. Reversal of the CD4 to CD8 ratio persisted for five years or more but returned to normal after six years. CD57+ CD16- cells were markedly increased from three months up to a maximum of five years after transplantation. CD57 is also known as HNK1, which is found in NK cells and T cells and B cell subsets. These cells were increased between three and six months after transplantation, irrespective of GVHD, but changes after one year or more differed among patients without GVHD and those with acute GVHD. The absolute number of CD57+ CD16- cells tend to gradually return to normal after one year or more in the group without GVHD but only after six years or more in patients with GVHD.

## LYMPHOKINE-ACTIVATED KILLER (LAK) CELLS

Another cell that has been proposed for the prevention of GVHD and which also expresses asialo $GM_1$ is the LAK cell. Data show that the LAK cells (enriched lymphokine-activated bone marrow, lymphokine-activated splenocytes and cloned LAK cells) can suppress mixed lymphocyte cultures (MLC). These LAK cells were able to prevent GVHD.[81] Data demonstrate that adoptive transfer of either donor type or recipient type LAK cells abrogated or inhibited the resistance of irradiated mice to allogeneic bone marrow or third party unrelated bone marrow. In addition to inhibiting allogeneic resistance, adoptive transfer of recipient type LAK cells prevents lethal GVHD and permits long-term engraftment of allogeneic bone marrow. There is evidence that LAK cells have two important functions: (1) veto activity, i.e., the ability to specifically prevent immune responses against their own self-surface antigen and (2) natural suppression, the ability of similar cells to nonspecifically suppress immune responses to both self- and non-self-antigens. Therefore, adoptive immunotherapy with LAK cells may be an interesting method to prevent graft rejection and GVHD in human BMT recipients. One important question is the relative contribution of recipient type versus donor type LAK cells. Donor type LAK cells appear to be more efficient inhibitors of allogeneic resistance than recipient type LAK cells; however, their use in bone marrow transplantation may be limited by their capacity to cause lethal GVHD. Yet adoptive transfer of MHC incompatible LAK cells does not necessarily cause GVHD in the irradiated recipients. Even repeated transfers (once every four days for three transfers) did not result in GVHD.[83] These data suggest that it is feasible to transfer allogeneic LAK cells, at least in murine models.

Because asialo $GM_1$ has been found on the surface of activated macrophages, it is important to distinguish between the two most likely targets for the in-vivo effect of anti-asialo $GM_1$. That is, whether this monoclonal antibody affects T cells or macrophages. When the effects of anti-asialo $GM_1$ antibodies are compared between alloantigen-stimulated T-cell proliferation versus antigen presentation, T-cell proliferation was markedly reduced by treatment with antibody whereas antigen presentation functioned normally. Therefore it appears that anti-asialo $GM_1$ prevents GVHD disease by reducing T-cell proliferation. This suggests that the prevention of GVHD does not directly involve NK cells or antigen presentation but rather activation of donor T cells.[84]

Finally, the route of injection may also affect the occurrence of GVHD.[85] Intraperitoneal injection of spleen cells from C57Bl/6 into completely allogeneic immunodeficient SCID mice induced GVHD, whereas intravenous injection of the same cells did not even though donor cells were present in the recipient spleens. These data suggest that the route of administration of these cells may lead to tolerance against host antigens.

# REFERENCE

1. Storb R, Deeg HJ, Pepe M et al. Methotrexate and cyclosporine versus cyclosporine alone for prophylaxis of graft-versus-host disease in patients given HLA-identical marrow grafts for leukemia: Long-term follow-up of a controlled trial. Blood 1989; 73: 1729.

2. Sullivan KM, Witherspoon R, Deeg HJ, Sanders JE, Shulman HM, Doney K, Appelbaum FR, Schubert MM, Stewart P, Springmeyer S, McDonald BG, Storb R, Thomas ED. Chronic graft-versus-host disease in man. In. Progress in Bone Marrow Transplantation. New York: Alan R. Liss, 1987: 473.

3. Forman SJ, Blume KG, Krance RA et al. A prospective randomized study of acute graft-v-host disease in 107 patients with leukemia: methotrexate/prednisone v cyclosporin a/prednisone. Transplant Proc 1987; 19: 2605.

4. Chao NJ, Schmidt G, Niland JC et al. Cyclosporine, methotrexate, and prednisone compared to cyclosporine and prednisone for prophylaxis of acute graft-versus-host disease. N Engl J Med 1993; 329:1225.

5. Vallera DA, Soderling CCB, Carlson GJ, Kersey JH. Bone marrow transplantation across major histocompatibility barriers in mice. Effect of elimination of T cells from donor grafts by treatment with monoclonal Thy-1.2 plus complement or antibody alone. Transplantation 1981; 31: 218.

6. Hamilton BL, Bevan MJ, Parkman R. Anti-recipient cytotoxic T lymphocyte precursors are present in the spleens of mice with acute graft-versus-host disease due to minor histocompatibility antigens. J Immunol 1981; 126: 621.

7. Piguet P. GVHR elicited by products of class I or class II loci of the MHC: Analysis of the response of mouse T lymphocytes to products of class I and class II loci of the MHC in correlation with GVHR-induced mortality, medullary aplasia, and enteropathy. J Immunol 1985; 135: 1353.

8. Grebe SC, Streilein JW. Graft-versus-host disease. Adv Immunol 1976; 22: 119.

9. Hale G, Cobbold SP, Waldman H. For Campath-1 Users: T-cell depletion with Campath-1 in allogeneic bone marrow transplantation. Transplantation 1988; 45: 753.

10. Ritz J, Soiffer R, Nadler LM et al. Prevention of rejection of genetically non-identical bone marrow grafts by total body irradiation prior to standard pre-transplant conditioning. Proc Am Soc Hematol 1988; 7: 1522.

11. Vallera DA, Ash R., Zanjani ED et al. Anti-T-cell reagents for human bone marrow transplantation: Ricin linked to three monoclonal antibodies. Science 1983; 22: 512.

12. O'Reilly RJ, Kapoor N, Kirkpatrick D et al. Transplantation for severe combined immunodeficiency using histocompatible parental marrow fractionated by soybean agglutinin and sheep red blood cells: Experience in six consecutive cases. Transplant Proc 1983; 15: 1431.

13. Kernan N., Flomenberg N, Dupont B, O'Reilly RJ. Graft rejection in recipients of T-cell-depleted HLA-nonidentical marrow transplants for leukemia. Transplantation 1987. 43: 842.

14. Eto M., Mayumi J, Tomita Y, Yoshikai Y, Nishimura Y, Maeda T, Ando T, Nomoto K. Specific destruction of host-reactive mature T cells of donor origin prevents graft-versus-host disease in cyclophosphammide induced tolerant mice. J Immunol 1991. 146: p. 1402-1409.

15. Martin P. The role of donor lymphoid cells in allogeneic marrow engraftment. Bone Marrow Transplant 1990; 6: 283.

16. Down J, Mauch P, Warhol M, Neben S, Ferrara J. The effect of donor T lymphocytes and total-body irradiation on hemopoietic engraftment and pulmonary toxicity following experimental allogeneic bone marrow transplantation. Transplantation 1992; 54: 802.

17. Dietrich PY, Caignard A, Diu A et al. Analysis of T-cell receptor variability in transplanted patients with acute graft-versus-host disease. Blood 1992; 80: 2419.

18. van Els C, Baker A, Zwinderman AH, Zwaan FE, van Rood JJ, Goulmy E. Effector mechanisms in graft-versus-host disease in response to minor histocompatibility antigens. II. Evidence of a possible involvement of proliferative T cells. Transplantation 1990; 50: 67.

19. Korngold R, Wettstein PJ. Immunodominance in the graft-versus-host disease T-cell response to minor histocompatibility antigens. J Immunol 1990; 145: 4079.

20. Irschick EU, Hladik F, Niederwieser D et al. Studies on the mechanism of tolerance or graft-versus-host disease in allogeneic bone marrow recipients at the level of cytotoxic T-cell precursor frequencies. Blood 1992; 79: 1622.

21. Niederwieser D, Grassegger A, Aubock J et al. Correlation of minor histocompatibility antigen-specific cytotoxic T lymphocytes with graft-versus-host disease status and analyses of tissue distribution of their target antigens. Blood 1993; 81: 2200.

22. Kaminski E, Sharrock C, Hows J et al. Frequency analysis of cytotoxic T lymphocyte precursors-possible relevance to HLA-matched unrelated donor bone marrow transplantation. Bone Marrow Transplant 1988; 3: 149.

23. Kaminski E, Hows J, Man S et al. Prediction of graft-versus-host disease by frequency analysis of cytotoxic T cells after unrelated donor bone marrow transplantation. Transplantation 1989 48: 608.

24. Eiermann T, Fakler J, Goldmann SF. The incidence of DPB1 differences between serological and mixed lymphocyte culture matched unrelated individuals: Implications for selection of bone marrow donors. Bone Marrow Transplant 1992; 9: 157.

25. De Bueger M, Bakker A, van Rood JJ, Goulmy E. Minor histocompatibility antigens, defined by graft-vs-host disease-derived cytotoxic T lymphocytes, show variable expression on human skin cells. Eur J Immunol 1991; 21: 2839.

26. Theobald M, Nierle T, Bunjes D, Arnold R, Heimpel H. Host-specific interleukin-2-secreting donor T-cell precursors as predictors of acute graft-versus-host disease in bone marrow transplantation between HLA-identical siblings. N Engl J Med 1992; 327:1613.

27. van Els C, Bakker A, Zwinderman AH, Zwaan FE, van Rood JJ, Goulmy E. Effector mechanisms in graft-versus-host disease in response to minor histocompatibility antigens. I. Absence of correlation with cytotoxic effector cells.

Transplantation 1990; 50: 62.

28. Johnsen HE, Bostrom L, Moller J, Jorgensen JA, Jensen L, Ringden O. A study of donor alloreactivity, which may predict acute graft-versus-host disease in HLA identical bone marrow transplantations for early leukemia. Scand J Immunol 1992; 35: 353.

29. Johnsen HE, Mickelson E, Beatty PG, Hansen JA. Donor alloreactivity may predict acute graft-versus host disease in patients receiving marrow transplants from HLA identical siblings. Bone Marrow Transpl 1992; 9: 91.

30. Kohn F, Sladek NE. Ex vivo treatment of murine splenocyte-supplemented bone marrow inocula with mafosfamide prior to allogeneic transplantation in an attempt to prevent lethal graft-versus-host disease without compromising engraftment. Immunopharmacol Immunotoxicol 1988; 10: 387.

31. Touraine J-L, Roncarolo M-G, Bacchetta R et al. Fetal liver transplantation: biology and clinical results. Bone Marrow Transplant 1993; 11 (Suppl 1):119.

32. Korngold R, Sprent J. T-cell subsets and graft-versus-host disease. Transplantation 1987; 44: 335.

33. Korngold R. Lethal graft-versus-host disease in mice directed to multiple minor histocompatibility antigens: Features of CD8[+] and CD4[+] T-cell responses. Bone Marrow Transpl 1992; 9: 355.

34. Sprent J, Schaefer M, Korngold R. Role of T-cell subsets in lethal graft-versus-host disease (GVHD) directed to class I versus class II H-2 differences. J Immunol 1990; 144: 2946.

35. Kelso A. Frequency analysis of lymphokine-secreting CD4[+] and CD8[+] T cells activated in a graft-versus-host reaction. J Immunol 1990; 145: 2167.

36. Klarnet JP, Kern DE, Dower SK, Matis LA, Cheever MA, Greenberg PD. Helper independent CD8[+] cytotoxic T lymphocytes express IL-1 receptors and require IL-1 for secretion of IL-2. J Immunol 1989; 142: 2187.

37. Mizuochi T, McKean D, Singer A. IL-1 as a co-factor for lymphokine secreting CD8[+] murine T cells. J Immunol 1988; 141: 1571.

38. Korngold R, Sprent J. Variable capacity of L3T4[+] T cells to cause lethal graft-versus-host disease across minor histocompatibility barriers in mice. J Exp Med 1987; 165: 1552

39. Janeway C, Yagi J, Conrad PJ et al. T-cell responses to Mls and to bacterial proteins that mimic its behavior. Immunol Rev 1989; 107: 61

40. Truitt RL, Atasoylu AA. Contribution of CD4[+] and CD8[+] T cells to graft-versus-host disease and graft-versus-leukemia reactivity after transplantation of MHC-compatible bone marrow. Bone Marrow Transpl 1991; 8: 51.

41. O'Kunewick J, Kociban DL, Buffo MJ. Comparative effects of various T-cell subtypes on GVHD in a murine model for MHC-matched unrelated donor transplant. Bone Marrow Transpl 1990; 5: 145.

42. Atkinson K, Cooley M, Farrelly H et al. T-4[+]cells can initiate human graft-versus-host disease. Transplant Proc 1987; 19: 2879.

43. Knulst AC, Bril-Bazuin C, Benner R. Prevention of lethal graft-vs.-host disease by a single low dose injection of anti-T-cell monoclonal antibody to the allograft recipients. Eur J Immunol 1991; 21: 103.

44. Damle NK, Mohagheghpur N, Hansen JA, Engleman EG. Alloantigen-specific cytotoxic and suppressor T lymphocytes are derived from phenotypically distinct precursors. J Immunol 1983; 131:2296.

45. Hall BM, Gurley K, Dorsch SE. The possible role of cytotoxic T cells in the mediation of first set allograft rejection. Transplantation 1985; 40: 336.

46. Pearce NW, Hall B, Dorsch SE. T-cell subsets mediating lethal graft-versus-host disease: Demonstration that synergy between CD4[+] and CD8[+] T cells is the predominant mechanism in low responder rat strains. Cell Immunol 1989; 122: 517.

47. Dorsch S, Roser B. T cells mediate transplantation tolerance. Nature 1975; 258: 237.

48. Nossal G. Cellular mechanisms of immunological tolerance. Annu Rev Immunol 1983; 1: 33.

49. Nossal GJV, Pike BL. Functional clonal deletion in immunological tolerance to major histocompatibility complex antigens. Proc Natl Acad Sci 1981; 78: 3844.

50. Norton J, Al-Saffar N, Sloane JP. An immunohistological study of $\gamma/\delta$ lymphocytes in human cutaneous graft-versus-host disease. Bone Marrow Transpl 1991; 7: 205.

51. Norton J, Al-Saffar N, Sloane JP. Immunohistological study of distribution of $\gamma/\delta$ lymphocytes after allogeneic bone marrow transplantation. J Clin Pathol 1992; 45: 1027.

52. O'Kunewick J, Meredith RF, Raikow RB, Brozovich BJ, Maglier K. Fatal response suggestive of graft-versus-host reaction following transplantation of splenic cells from allogeneic athymi (nude) donor. Transplantation 1981; 31: 201.

53. O'Kunewick J, Beschorner WE, Buffo MJ, Kociban DL. Histopathology of a possible graft-versus-host reaction induced by nude mouse spleen cells. Transplantation 1985; 39: 447.

54. Hamilton BL, Parkman R. Kinetics of the anti-recipient cytotoxic cell response of mice with minor antigen-graft-vs-host disease. J Immunol 1982; 128: 376

55. Lapidot T, Factorowich Y, Lubin I, Reisner Y. Enhancement of T-cell-depleted bone marrow allografts in the absence of graft-versus-host disease is mediated by CD8[-] CD4[+] thymocytes. Blood 1992; 80: 2406.

56. Uenaka A, Miemo M, Kuribayashi K, Shiku H, Nakayama E. Effector cells of lethal graft-versus-host disease (GVHD) in nude mice. Transpl Proc 1989; 21: 3031

57. Dokhelar M-C, Wiels J, Lipinski M et al. Natural killer cell activity in human bone marrow recipients: early appearance of peripheral natural killer activity in graft-versus-host disease. Transplantation 1981; 31: 61.

58. Acevedo A, Aramburu J, Lopez J et al. Identification of natural killer (NK) cells in lesions of human cutaneous graft-versus-host disease: Expression of a novel NK-associated surface antigen (Kp43) in mononuclear infiltrates. J Invest Dermatol 1991; 97: 659.

59. Roy C, Ghayur T, Kongshavn PAL, Lapp WS. Natural killer activity by spleen, lymph node, and thymus cells during the graft-versus-host reaction. Transplantation 1982; 34: 144.

60. Clancy J Jr, Mauser L, Chapman AL. Level and temporal pattern of naturally cytolytic cells during acute graft-versus-host disease (GVHD) in the rat. Cell Immunol 1983; 79: 1.

61. Ferrara J, Guillen FJ, van Dijken, PJ, Marion, A,Murphy, GF, Burakoff, SJ. Evidence that large granular lymphocyte of donor origin mediate acute graft-versus-host disease. Transplantation 1989; 47: 50.

62. Charley MR, Mikael A, Bennett M, Gilliam JN, Sontheimer RD. Prevention of lethal, minor determinant graft-vs-host disease in mice by the in vivo administration of anti-asialo $GM_1$. J Immunol 1983; 39: 85.

63. Cipriano D, Faanes R, Merluzzi VJ. Protection of mice against acute lethal graft-verus-host disease by treatment with anti-asialo GM1 antibody. Transplantation 1988; 47: 922.

64. Ghayur T, Seemayer T, Lapp W. Prevention of murine graft-versus-host disease by inducing and eliminating ASGM1[+] cells of donor origin. Transplantation 1988; 45: 586.

65. MacDonald GC, Gartner JG. Natural Killer (NK) cell activity in mice with acute graft-versus-host reactions: characterization of a Thy1[+] NK-like cell with a broadened spectrum of lytic activity in the spleen and lymph nodes. Scand J Immunol 1991; 33: 553.

66. MacDonald GC, Gartner JG. The host/donor origin of cells mediating NK and NK-like cytotoxic activity in $F_1$-hybrid mice with acute graft-versus-host disease. Transplantation 1991; 52: 141.

67. MacDonald GC, Gartner JG. Prevention of acute lethal graft-versus-host disease in F1 hybrid mice by pretreatment of the graft with anti-NK-1.1 and complement. Transplantation 1992; 54: 147.

68. Blazar BR, Soderling C, Koo GC, Vallera DA. Absence of a facilitory role for NK 1.1-positive donor cells in engraftment across a major histocompatibility barrier in mice. Transplantation 1988; 45: 876.

69. Levitsky HI, Golumbek P, Pardoll DM. The fate of CD4[-]8[-] T-cell receptor $\alpha\beta^+$ thymocytes. J Immunol 1991; 146: 1113.

70. Yankelevich B, Knobloch C, Nowicki M, Dennert G. A novel cell type responsible for marrow graft rejection in mice: T cells with NK phenotype cause acute rejection of marrow grafts. J Immunol 1989; 142:3423.

71. Johnson BD, Truitt R. A decrease in graft-versus-host disease without loss of graft-versus-leukemia reactivity after MHC-matched bone marrow transplantation by selective depletion of donor NK cells in vivo. Transplantation 1992; 54: 104.

72. Ferrara J, Marion A, Murphy G, Burakoff S. Acute graft-versus-host disease: pathogenesis and prevention with a monoclonal antibody in vivo. Transplant Proc 1987; 19: 2662.

73. Slavin S, Fuks Z, Kaplan HS et.al. Transplantation of allogeneic bone marrow without graft-versus-host disease using total lymphoid irradiation. J Exp Med 1978; 147: 963.

74. De Ruysscher D, Sobis H, Vandeputte M, Waer M. A subpopulation of asialo GM1-positive cells plays a protective role in the occurrence of graft-versus-host disease (GVHD) in mice. Transpl Proc 1991; 23: 804.

75. Strober S, Dejbashch-Jones S, Van Vlasselaer P et al. Cloned natural suppressor cell lines express the CD3+ CD4- CD8- surface phenotype and the alpha, beta heterodimer of the T cell antigen receptor. J Immunol 1989; 143: 1118.

76. De Ruysscher D, Dejbashch-Jones S, Vandeputte M, Waer M. A subset of asialo GM1[+] cells play a protective role in the occurrence of graft-versus-host disease in mice. J Immunol 1991; 146: 4065.

77. Dorshkind K, Rosse C. Physical, biologic and phenotypic properties of natural regulatory cells in murine bone marrow. Am J Anat 1982; 164: 1.

78. Strober S, Hertel-Wuff B, Schwadron RB. Role of natural suppressor cells in bone marrow transplantation. Transplant Proc 1987; 6: 88.

79. Sykes M, Eisenthal A, Sachs DH. Mechanism of protection from graft-versus-host disease in murine mixed allogeneic chimeras. J Immunol 1988; 140: 2903.

80. Kasai M, Yoneda T, Habu S, Maruyama Y, Okumura K, Tokunage T. In vivo effect of anti-asialo GM1 antibody on natural killer activity. Nature 1981; 291: 334.

81. Azuma E, Yamamoto H, Kaplan J. Use of lymphokine-activated keller cells to prevent bone marrow graft rejection and lethal graft-versus-host disease. J Immunol 1989; 143: 1524.

82. Fukuda H, Nakamura H, Tominaga N et al. Marked increase of CD57+CD16− cells in long-term survivors of graft-versus-host disease after allogeneic bone marrow transplantation. Jpn J Clin Oncol 1992; 22: 238.

83. Toshitani A, Taniguchi K, Himeno K, Kawano Y, Nomoto K. Adoptive transfer of H-2-incompatible lymphokine-activated killer (LAK) cells: An approach for successful cancer immunotherapy free from graft-versus-host disease (GVHD) using murine models. Cell Immunol 1988; 115: 373.

84. Charley MR, Mikhael A, Hackett J, Kumar V, Bennet M. Mechanism of anti-asialo GM$_1$ prevention of graft-vs-host disease: Identification of allo-antigen-activated T cells. J Invest Dermatol 1988; 91: 202-

85. Claesson MH, Rudolphi A, Tscherning T, Reimann J. CD3+ T cells in severe combined immunodeficiency (scid) mice IV: Graft-vs-host resistance of H-2d SCID mice to intravenous injection of allogeneic H-2b (C57BL/6) spleen cells. Eur J Immunol 1991; 21: 2057.

# CHAPTER 4

# MINOR HISTOCOMPATIBILITY ANTIGENS

## INTRODUCTION

In a previous chapter, we dealt with major histocompatibility antigens. These antigens are able to trigger T-cell responses specifically occurring after transplantation. Other antigens, however, such as ABO blood groups and related antigens can also provoke antibody-mediated graft rejection but are excluded from the usual tissue histocompatibility definition because they do not elicit T-cell responses. As the congenic strains of mice evolved, it became clear that other antigens were also important in triggering graft rejection. These less potent antigens are called minor histocompatibility antigens. This is somewhat of a misnomer: some of these "minor" histocompatibility antigens are neither weak nor minor and can trigger severe GVHD. However, we know very little about minor histocompatibility antigens. There is little information about the precise structure and chemical nature of these minor histocompatibility antigens. These antigens are critical in such transplantation as a matched sibling allogeneic bone marrow graft. It is clear that these minor histocompatibility antigens contribute to the definition of self versus non-self and are critical in establishing the T-cell repertoire in each individual.[1]

Use of congenic strains of mice helped to identify minor histocompatibility antigens. The total number of such minor histocompatibility antigen loci is not known but may be as few as 50 and as many as several hundred.[2,3] Over 40 minor histocompatibility differences are found between just two strains of mice. Moreover, linkage studies demonstrate that minor histocompatibility antigens are scattered throughout the genome. MHC restriction is a fundamental characteristic of minor histocompatibility antigen recognition.[4] Thus immune responses to minor histocompatibility antigens are strictly T-cell mediated, MHC-restricted and show features of antigen competition. This suggests that minor histocompatibility antigens are small peptides.

Further testing, using T-cell clones as genetic probes, demonstrated that T helper cells and CTLs specific for antigens, thought to be included by the same minor histocompatibility locus, were actually responding to products of separate but closely linked genes.[5] This suggested that genes defined by the reactivity of these T helper cells and CTLs are organized randomly throughout the genome relative to each other. Thus, a classic minor histocompatibility locus characterized by reproducible allograft rejection and CTL generation is likely to be a complex genetic unit in which many genes defined by CTL reactivity and T helper cell reactivity link closely to give the illusion that they segregate as a single unit. These minor histocompatibility genes and coproducts that selectively stimulate cytotoxic T cells are difficult to detect because of the need for coincident helper stimulus. A model has been proposed where minor histocompatibility genes and coproducts stimulate T helper cell reactivity but will not constitute an effective transplantation barrier.[6] There has been considerable controversy as to how many self gene products are found on MHC proteins as part of self proteins. For comparison, up to 88 allograft-defined minor histocompatibility antigens have been estimated among different mouse strains.[7] However, it is likely that many of these peptides are polymorphic, generating even larger numbers of potential minor histocompatibility loci. It is conceivable in this model that immune responses to environmental stimuli such as viruses or other infectious processes may provide a help stimulus for the generation of CTLs to these minor histocompatibility antigens. The literature suggests a contaminated environment results in a higher frequency of minor histocompatibility changes compared to a clean environment.[8] These environmental pathogens may stimulate T helper cells to support the generation of CTLs.

The nature of the antigenic stimulus for GVHD, i.e., "minor" histocompatibility antigens, and precise effector mechanisms remains to be defined. The damage caused by GVHD may be secondary to natural killer or "natural killer-like" cells, cytotoxic T cells, or through the release of a variety of lymphokines (IL-2, interferon, TNF, etc.). Seminal work done by Zinkernagel and Doherty demonstrated that T cells do not recognize antigens alone, but only in conjunction with the MHC of the presenting cells (presumably always self).[9] The MHC molecule, with a single cleft where binding occurs, acts as a receptor for the antigens. This complex is then recognized by the T-cell receptor.

In the past, it was generally accepted that individual MHC molecules were entirely homogeneous. The high frequency of T cells responding to foreign MHC molecules was perplexing. It seems now that the MHC molecules found on the cell surface associated with a variety of self peptides are, in fact, heterogeneous. Thus, alloreactivity could reflect recognition by the T-cell receptor of different peptides carried by the recipient MHC rather than the MHC molecules themselves.[10] These different peptides could represent the "minor" histocompatibility antigens. These alloreactive cells recognize self-peptide presented by recipient MHC and the peptide could be selected or shaped by the MHC molecule. Evidence for this comes from chimeric mouse class I molecules made by recombination of $K^d$ and $D^d$ sequences where $K^d$ specificity for the foreign antigen rests in residues 152, 155 and 156.[10-14] These are the same residues involved in most anti-$K^d$ allo-CTL clones, suggesting identical mechanisms for recognition of foreign antigen and allorecognition. Healy et al have generated HLA-A2/-A3 chimeric molecules and found that residues 114-116 and 152 are essential for the recognition of influenza antigens and that these residues are required for most allo-CTLs.[15]

T-cell antigens are peptides which can bind the MHC. Unanue and Babbitt et al first demonstrated, by equilibrium dialysis, that the lysozyme peptide 46-61 binds to I-A$^k$ but not to I-A$^d$.[16,17] Buus et al also demonstrated that ovalbumin peptide 323-339 could bind I-A$^d$ but not I-E$^d$, I-A$^k$ or I-E$^k$, and that Ia-peptide complexes could be separated by exclusion chromatography.[18,19] These complexes formed slowly (over approximately 24 hours), but once formed, were very stable. Biotin-labeled peptides confirmed this selective binding.[20] Other competition experiments complement the direct binding data, suggesting that class II molecules bind only one peptide at a time.[18,20-24] Buus et al studied the direct binding of 12 peptides to purified I-A$^d$, I-E$^d$, I-A$^k$ and I-E$^k$. Each peptide was found to bind to its functional restricted MHC molecule. Lambda repressor peptide 12-26, while its restriction element is I-A$^d$, bound strongly to I-E$^d$, suggesting that peptides can bind without eliciting a T-cell response. These "holes" in the T-cell repertoire presumably indicate that the lambda repressor resembles a self peptide presented by I-E$^d$, therefore leading to tolerance.[25] Various peptide analogs have been systematically studied and dissected into two groups of residues: those involved in binding to the presenting class II molecule and those that are recognized by the T-cell receptor.[26-29]

Viral proteins have been the major source of peptides for examining MHC class I and peptide interactions. For example, two peptides (50-63; 365-380) derived from the influenza nucleoprotein are restricted by H-2K$^k$ and H-2D$^b$.[30,31] These peptides bind directly onto histocompatibility molecules at a 1:1 ratio. The X-ray crystallographic data obtained by Bjorkman et al with the MHC class I molecule have confirmed this.[32] There is an antigen-binding pocket consisting of eight strands of β sheet forming a floor bounded by two α helical segments.[10,33] More recently, the structure of the class II antigen has also been elucidated and is similar to that of the class I molecule.[34]

A large body of data suggests that MHC molecules are associated with a variety of peptides from internal self proteins or internalized self proteins.

1. Antigen-presenting cells present the self allelic form of liver F protein.[35]
2. Schwann cells present myelin basic protein to T cells if induced by gamma interferon.[36]
3. There is binding of a self-lysozyme to mouse class II molecules and mouse lysozyme self peptide 46-62 can compete in vivo for T-cell activation by foreign antigens.[37,38]
4. Self hemoglobin-Ia complex exists in vivo on a variety of antigen-presenting cells.[39]
5. Syngeneic immunoglobulin fragments are presented by class II MHC molecules in vitro.[40-42]
6. Some peptides derived from self class I MHC molecules can be presented by self class II MHC molecules of the same individual and vice-versa.[24]
7. Coinjection of mouse lysozyme prevents priming of hen egg white lysozyme in mice.[43]
8. Reactions against minor transplantation antigens are MHC restricted and self-tolerance is MHC restricted, suggesting that some of the presented peptides are derived from polymorphic self peptides.[44,45]

9.  Finally, elution and sequencing of peptides bound to the MHC in
    mice demonstrates that these peptides are derived from endogenous
    proteins.[46,47]

Thus, a major target of acute GVHD in HLA-matched bone marrow
transplantation (from the point of view of the incoming T-cell) are the
"self" MHC class II molecules plus non-self peptides. The nature of minor
transplantation antigens includes any amino acid sequence polymorphism
in any self protein that might differ between donor and host even among
MHC identical donor-host combinations. This concept, and the concurrent
concepts of the mechanisms of antigen presentation to these T cells, the
nature of the peptide antigens presented to these T cells and the recognition
of the peptide MHC complex by the T-cell receptor have been considerably
clarified in the past five years.

Evidence that the minor histocompatibility antigens are peptides in the
self MHC-binding groove has been elegantly demonstrated by Fischer-Lindahl
et al.[48-50] Her work describes a maternally-transmitted antigen, Mtα, which
is a mouse histocompatibility antigen. It consists of Mtf (maternally transmitted factor), a peptide from the mitochondrial encoded ND1 protein (a
subunit of NADH dehydrogenase) and HMT, a $\beta_2$ microglobulin-associ-
ated restriction element for cytotoxic T lymphocytes. Expression of Mtα
depends on HMT, an MHC-linked class I-like gene, $\beta_2$ microglobulin and
Mtf. The sequence analysis of the entire mitochondrion genomes from
three strains that differ in Mtf ($\beta$,$\gamma$,$\delta$) was compared to the common form
(Mtf$^\alpha$). Only a single amino acid was different in the four genomes, affecting amino acid residue 6 of ND1. Moreover, incubation of non-Mtf$^\alpha$ target
cells with synthetic peptide ND1α 1-17 (the first 17 amino acids of the
ND1 protein of Mtf$^\alpha$ mice) rendered them susceptible to lysis by Mtf$^\alpha$-
specific cytotoxic T cells. The same result was obtained using non-Mtf$^\beta$
target cells which were lysed by Mtf$^\beta$ specific cytotoxic T cells after incubation with the allelic form ND1 $\beta$ 1-17. These data demonstrate that (1) a
peptide binding to the MHC molecule forms a target for CTLs; (2) the
binding is MHC-restricted and (3) a single variation of one amino acid
residue caused changes in the antigen binding and recognition by CTLs.
Therefore, Mtf variations are a result of a single residue difference of the
ND1 peptide, and such peptides function as histocompatibility antigens.

A minor histocompatibility antigen has been both molecularly and
functionally defined, in a study which took advantage of the allelic differences in structurally characterized intracellular myxovirus-resistance protein
(Mx) and investigated its antigenicity.[51] Skin grafts from congenic Mx$^+$
mice carried the functional Mx1 gene and were rejected by mice lacking
functional Mx1 gene (Mx$^-$). Cytotoxic MHC class I-restricted effector T cells
specific for the Mx protein and the H2$^k$ antigen were strongly induced in
the Mx$^-$ mice immunized with spleen cells from interferon treated Mx$^+$
mice. The nuclear Mx protein is a product of the $\alpha\beta$ interferon-regulated
gene Mx1 that confers resistance to the influenza virus. This particular
study investigated the antigenicity of this Mx protein based on the hypothesis that minor histocompatibility antigens are allelic forms of MHC class I-
restricted self antigen recognized by the cytotoxic T cells. The investigators
assumed that these minor histocompatibility antigens are internal cell

antigens that are processed and then presented by MHC class I protein similar to viral antigens. They were able to show that skin from Mx$^+$ mice was rejected slowly and incompletely by congenic Mx$^-$ transplant recipients. Fragments of this protein were recognized on the cell surface of target cells by the restricted murine T cells (H2$^k$). This agrees with the proposal by Fisher-Lindahl's suggestion that minor histocompatibility antigens are self-components presented by the MHC antigens. These results also corroborate the experiments by Townsend et al has demonstrating that viral antigen fragments presented by the MHC class I molecule are recognized by the cytotoxic T cells.[31]

The concentration of peptide and the MHC complex on the cell surface is probably very important for the activation of T cells. Quantitative limitations may explain why many self products are nonimmunogenic minor histocompatibility antigens.[9] Most self molecules or self peptides are processed but their concentration may be too low to successfully compete for binding of MHC molecules.[38] Thus, high levels of a particular peptide, in this case Mx expression, may be necessary and critical for recognition by the cytotoxic T lymphocytes. Additional support comes from the observation that higher expression of the Mx protein correlates with greater susceptibility to Mx-specific cytotoxic T cells. Therefore the two examples above are compatible with the concept that self antigens are expressed at relatively high concentrations and associated with MHC molecules to be immunogenic and recognized by CTLs. These data are also compatible with the need of self antigens to be (1) expressed in relatively high concentrations, (2) associated with the MHC molecules at a sufficiently high rate and (3) presented as minor histocompatibility antigens.

## IMMUNE INTERVENTION

This molecular trio, composed of a peptide, the MHC molecule and the T-cell receptor (TcR), has become a target of immune intervention in autoimmune diseases.[52] Injection of monoclonal antibodies directed against MHC class II molecule can block various experimental autoimmune diseases such as systemic lupus erythematosus (SLE) and experimental autoimmune encephalomyelitis (EAE).[53,54] However, anti-Ia monoclonal antibodies cause prolonged B-cell depletion.[55] Recently anti-TcR antibodies have prevented disease induction or the reversal of disease in EAE but, as a general rule, most autoimmune diseases probably do not have the limited heterogeneity of TcR usage as EAE.[56,57]

The use of a peptide as an immunomodulator is an attractive approach. Since there is only one cleft per MHC molecule where peptide binding can occur, it is possible to obtain high affinity peptides which will bind to disease-associated MHC molecules without the activation of disease-causing T cells. Wraith et al demonstrated that such peptides could be designed.[52] Substitution experiments demonstrated that myelin basic protein (MBP) Ac1-11[4A] (substituted alanine at position 4) resulted in enhanced response of a T-cell hybridoma (1934.4), which faithfully reproduces the pattern of recognition shown for the majority of T-cell clones responsive to MBP. Subsequent substitution of alanine at position 3 (Ac1-11[3A]) or position 6 (Ac1-11[6A]) resulted in no response. This lack of response was not due to lack of the binding of the peptide to I-A$^u$ as determined by the ability of peptide analogs to compete with a photoaffinity probe for binding to I-A$^u$.

This information led to the design of peptides that bound to the MHC, yet did not cross-react with the autoantigen. The peptide analog (Ac 1-11[4A]) was shown to be heteroclitic for MHC binding. This same peptide is not immunogenic for encephalitogenic T cells in vivo. Since self peptides must bind to MHC molecules in order to activate the T cells responsible for autoimmune disease, the activation of auto-aggressive T cells in EAE might be inhibited by "blocking" peptides which compete for the binding of self peptides to class II MHC molecules. Ac 1-11[4A] inhibits disease that is induced by the autoantigen itself, although in this model inhibition may occur through other methods besides competition for MHC binding.

Lamont et al demonstrated the inhibition of EAE in SJL/J mice by using a peptide sequence unrelated to the disease-inducing peptide, but with high affinity for I-A$^s$ molecules.[58,59] Several criteria were used to select the inhibiting peptide. First, the peptide was shown to bind to I-A$^s$ by the inhibition of antigen presentation in vitro to an I-A$^s$-restricted T-cell hybridoma. Second, the peptide was relatively resistant to proteases, a property known to enhance inhibition by peptides.[58] A peptide (KM-core extension), based on the antigenic core sequence of ovalbumin 323-339 and bound strongly to I-A$^s$, was resistant to serum proteases and was highly effective in inhibiting EAE induced with the encephalitogenic peptide. The control peptide HEL 46-61, which does not bind to I-A$^s$, had no effect on EAE induction. Therefore, KM-core functioned as a MHC "blocking" peptide.

These peptides could effectively block donor T-cell recognition of host "self". We predict that in HLA identical BMT (as with human HLA-matched sibling transplants), the occurrence of GVHD results from host peptides which are different and therefore foreign to the donor T cells, analogous to Mtf described by Fischer-Lindahl as discussed above. That is, the donor T cells, in this case murine PL/J or SJL/J T cells, will recognize the B10.PL or B10.S MHC molecule as self, as they are MHC-identical. However, the B10 self peptides bound to the B10.PL or B10.S MHC molecule are different from the PL/J or SJL/J self peptides, respectively. These host peptides are sufficient to induce activation of donor T cells and can cause GVHD. Use of selected peptides that bind avidly to the host MHC class II displace endogenous host peptides. The use of specific peptides with well-defined functional residues may allow the determination of what causes GVHD in a MHC-matched BMT. Our hypothesis was that prevention of recognition of these molecules (minor histocompatibility antigens) is sufficient to prevent or ameliorate GVHD.

The design for these studies is demonstrated in Figures 4.1 and 4.2. Ac1-11, AcASQKRPSQRHG, the acetylated N-terminal 1-11 peptide of myelin basic protein (MBP) and its analogs have been well-characterized. Previous studies of the role of individual residues of Ac 1-11 in vitro showed that residue 4 influences binding of the peptide to I-A$^u$, whereas residues 3 and 6 are important T-cell interaction residues. Substitution of alanine for lysine normally found at residue 4 creates the peptide analog, Ac 1-11[4A], AcASQARPSQRHG, which binds 10- to 100-fold better to I-A$^u$ than the normal peptide.[52] Ac 1-11[4A] is nonimmunogenic and nonencephalitogenic in vivo and prevents EAE when administered before or at the time of immunization with Ac 1-11 or even at the time of disease onset. Ac1-11[4A] was, therefore, chosen as a binding peptide for I-A$^u$. The epitope 35-47 of MBP (TGILDSIGRFFSG), which is recognized in association with I-E$^u$ molecules, was chosen as a binding peptide for I-E$^u$. The KM core extension peptide, KMKMVHAAHAKMKM, based on the antigenic core sequence of ovalbumin 323-339 binds strongly to I-A$^s$, is resistant to serum

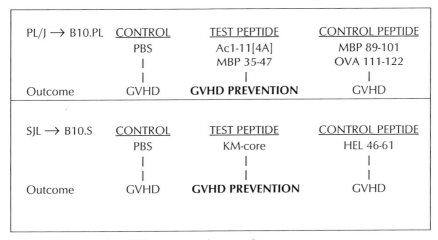

Fig. 4.1. Schematic design of experimental protocol.

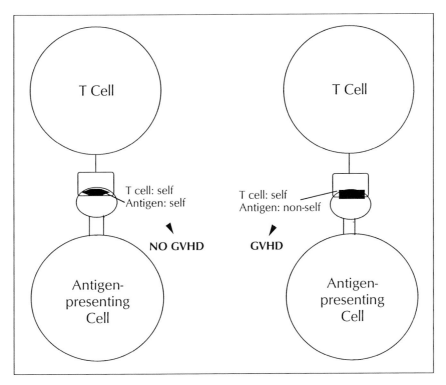

Fig. 4.2. Diagram of proposed interaction between self and non-self peptides with the same MHC molecules found in the host and the recipients of MHC-matched sibling/donor pairs. Note that the presence of non-self peptides bound to the MHC molecules will trigger the T cell.

proteases and is highly effective in inhibiting EAE induced in SJL mice by proteolipid protein (PLP) 139-151.[58,59] SJL mice express I-A$^s$ but do not express I-E$^s$.

After transplantation, peptides were injected intraperitoneally (IP) daily for the first three weeks. The frequency of injections was tapered to three times per week for two weeks and two times per week for two weeks and then stopped. Control mice received either phosphate-buffered saline (PBS) or a nonbinding control peptide (MBP 89-101: VHFFKNIVTPRTP, for I-A$^u$ and I-E$^u$ or HEL 46-61: NTDGSTDYGILQINSR, for I-A$^s$). Mice were followed for 100 days after bone marrow transplantation for histological changes and proteinuria as indicators of GVHD. Skin biopsies were sampled on day 30, while on peptide therapy, and on day 70 (21 days after peptide therapy had been discontinued). Histology was examined by two independent observers, and the changes were quantitated.

Data pooled from two identical experiments demonstrated that the incidence of histologic GVHD on day 30 (Fig. 4.3) was 16/16 in both groups B (PBS) and C (nonbinding peptide), and 0/14 in syngeneic controls (Group D). GVHD was considered as prevented in an individual mouse if both the number of epidermal dyskeratotic cells/mm skin and the number of vacuolated cells/mm skin were decreased by at least 80% com-

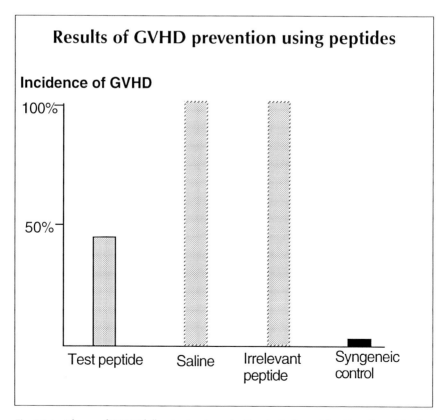

Fig. 4.3. Incidence of GVHD following treatment with selected peptides. Use of peptides that bound to class II antigens prevented GVHD in nearly 60% of the animals. In contrast, saline or a peptide that did not bind to the class II molecule failed to prevent GVHD.

pared to positive (mean of group B) and negative background controls (mean of group D). No prevention was found with the nonbinding peptide MBP 89-101 (n=16). However, in 10/18 mice (55.6 %) that received Ac 1-11[4A] and MBP 35-47 (Group A), GVHD was prevented (p<0.001). The histologic appearance was surprisingly clear-cut, suggesting that GVHD prevention is likely to be an all or nothing effect. Furthermore, the effect of the binding peptides was at least in part transient, since 4/18 mice in group A developed histologic evidence of GVHD after discontinuation of the "therapeutic peptide" when tested 70 days posttransplant (Fig. 4.3). Thus, the overall rate of prevention on day 70 was 33.3%.

Chimerism was tested in two of the four described experiments using skin grafts from donor mice. Skin grafts were performed on all transplanted animals on day 100 and followed for rejection or acceptance for another 50 days. In the PL/J → B10.PL system, 4 of 12 mice in group A had not shown GVHD on day 70. Three of these four mice did not reject their skin grafts, indicating that they were chimeras, and that GVHD "prevention" was not related to regrowth of autologous bone marrow. One of these four mice died on day 108 and could not be evaluated. These skin graft results demonstrate that there is prevention of GVHD rather than rejection of the allogeneic cells and recovery of autologous bone marrow.

A second bone marrow transplantation model was chosen in order to determine whether the above results were a unique property of the peptides Ac 1-11[4A] and MBP 35-47 and the particular murine strain combination or whether a similar mechanism might operate in other strain combinations as well. KM-core extension peptide was chosen for its well-characterized, high binding affinity and resistance to serum proteases. Experimental mice that received KM-core peptide demonstrated significantly less epidermal dyskeratotic cells/mm skin and vacuolated cells/mm skin than their controls. Data pooled from two identical experiments showed that the incidence of GVHD on day 30 was 15/15 and 13/13 in control groups compared to 11/16 (68.8%) in mice that were treated with KM-core (p<0.05).

The results of four experiments demonstrate that peptides with high binding affinity for the class II MHC molecules can be used to prevent GVHD in two murine models of graft-versus-host disease across minor histocompatibility barriers. The effect seems to be transient in some mice and permanent in others. The precise mechanisms by which Ac 1-11[4A], 35-47 and KM-core prevent GVHD need to be explained further. The experiments described here suggest the possibility of a transient effect caused by competitive binding of Ac 1-11 [4A] to I-A$^u$ and of MBP 35-47 to I-E$^u$, or of KM-core to I-A$^s$, but do not rule out the activation of suppressive or regulatory cells. Immunodominance of the test peptides could also explain some of these observations. However, no immune response to any of these peptides (MBP: Ac 1-11[4A], 35-47 or 89-101) was detected three to four weeks following total body irradiation and bone marrow transplantation in the PL/J → B10.PL system. Finally, although class I molecules were not targeted, 10 times fewer cells are necessary to establish GVHD in congenic strains differing in the class II region compared to differences in class I region. Moreover, GVHD in man is more prominent when the donor-recipient pairs are mismatched in the DR region.

We suggest that the high affinity peptides which are known to bind to the class II molecules displace endogenous peptides and thus down modulate allogeneic T-cell recognition of other minor histocompatibility antigens (other endogenous peptides) in the recipient. Thus, use of the test peptide known to bind to the MHC class II molecule results in a significant decrease in GVHD. Use of another peptide that does not bind to the class II molecule does not result in protection from the development of GVHD. The similar results in two separate murine models, using completely different peptides, demonstrate that peptide binding to class II MHC molecules allows for down modulation and prevention of murine GVHD.

Following bone marrow transplantation in humans, anti-host T-cell reaction is directed against several minor histocompatibility antigens presented by MHC class I and class II molecules. Sixteen patients were studied with anti-host T-cell responses.[60] T cells isolated from patients' peripheral blood demonstrated significantly higher anti-host proliferation in patients with acute GVHD than those without acute GVHD. These proliferative responses could be blocked by monoclonal antibodies against HLA DR but not by monoclonal antibodies against HLA-A,B,C, HLA-DQ or DP. These findings suggest that anti-host T-cell responses activated during the acute phase of GVHD are directed against minor histocompatibility antigens. This response is mediated by CD4+ cells and uses the HLA-DR molecule as a common restriction element for this minor antigen presentation. It is interesting that HLA-DR is strongly induced on keratinocytes and enterocytes in acute GVHD.[61-63] Therefore these antigens could act as presenting cells leading to the occurrence of acute GVHD. A different observation is made in the nodal tissues. Using immunoperoxidase techniques to stain T-cell subsets in frozen sections of lymph nodes, there was a reversal of CD4+ to CD8+ ratios in 46% of the patients with acute GVHD compared to only 13% of those patients without GVH.[64] These data demonstrate that abnormal intranodal CD4:CD8 ratios are present more frequently in patients with GVHD. This abnormal CD4:CD8 ratio may add to the dysfunctional B-cell maturation.

Most of the data presented in these discussions will be limited to matched related sibling BMT. In cases of matched unrelated donor transplantation, the risk of GVHD will be significantly higher due to the disparity for the multiple minor, and possibly major, histocompatibility antigens. The two concepts involved in the increased response may be related to the strength or type of the antigen. Under these circumstances, it may be that CD4+ and CD8+ T cells recognize the donor histocompatibility molecules much more strongly than other types of antigen. The first theory, then, is the antigen density theory. When a matched unrelated donor transplanted T cell sees an antigen-presenting cell with a foreign MHC class II molecule on it, every single class II molecule on the surface of that antigen-presenting cell is foreign to the T cell and every class II molecule may look different unless they are genotypically matched. Alternatively, on an antigen-presenting cell with "self" molecules, such as a peptide of tetanus or other self peptides, maybe only 1 of 100, 1 of 1,000, or 1 of 10,000 of the MHC class II molecules has a modified determinant so that by antigen density, the fully allogeneic MHC mismatched antigen-presenting cell contains 100- to 1,000-fold more novel antigens on its surface.

Antigen density is not only important in MHC expression but also in the expression of any antigen. Another example of the importance of antigen density is the evidence that reduced Thy1 expression in Thy1.1 mice prevents suppression of GVHD with anti-Thy1 monoclonal antibodies.[65] Thus a rat anti-Thy1 monoclonal antibody suppresses GVHD in a fully mismatched donor/recipient combination. When Thy1.1 mice were used as donors, this did not occur. This is because Thy1.2 mice have practically all T cells expressing both Thy1 and the T-cell marker Ly1. In contrast, there exists in Thy1.1 mice a population of Thy1$^-$, Ly1$^+$ T cells. Using quantitative immunofluorescence, it was determined that Thy1 antigen binding sites in Thy1$^+$ cells from Th 1.1 mice were considerably fewer compared to those of Thy1.2 mice. Thus, a monoclonal antibody against anti-Thy1 may have variable effects, which may also partially explain why such an approach has not been uniformly successful in humans.

An alternative is the antigen frequency hypothesis. This hypothesis suggests that the allogeneic MHC molecules are all on the donor cell surface presenting a variety of different peptides. Many of these are autologous peptides such as peptides of albumin. If those serum albumin peptides are being presented by self MHC molecules, they form a determinant to which the self T cells are tolerant. But if those same peptides are presented by an allogeneic MHC molecule, it creates a allogeneic determinant. The result is that every allogeneic MHC antigen is not only different from self but also different from every other. There may be dozens of different determinants even though there is only a single allogeneic MHC difference.

## NON-MHC GENES IN GHVD

By using genetic analysis in a specific murine model, some investigators suggested that one autosomal locus (non-H-2 gene) is responsible for the differences in GVHD response of the mouse strains DBA/2J and DBA/2Ha cells. The presence of the DBA/2Ha allele is dominant.[66] The different GVHD responses were found to be regulated by a radiosensitive recipient mechanism responding to the DBA/2J donor cells. These data also suggest that an Lyt2 recipient cell plays a role in this mechanism. It appears that donor cells express an antigen that induces the recipient response. In a similar model, injection of C57Bl/6 spleen cells into unirradiated (C57Bl/6 x DBA/2) F1 hybrid recipient mice results in an acute form of GVHD characterized by CTL, suppressor cells and runting. In contrast, an injection of DBA/2 spleen cells into the same recipients results in a chronic form of GVHD which is characterized by a lack of CTL and hypoproduction of immunoglobulins and auto antibodies. This difference appears to be restricted to a single locus of graft-versus-host reaction on chromosome 7 which controls whether acute or chronic GVHD results.

Another study suggested the possibility of a gene distal to the HLA-A gene in the etiology of GVHD in humans.[67] The data support the hypothesis that mismatching for immune response genes near but distal to HLA-A may contribute to acute GVHD. However, it is not likely that this would be a single locus since multiple minor histocompatibility antigens are important in acute GVHD. It is likely that such studies identify proteins and their subsequent peptide fragments that are presented by class I or class II MHC molecules. These peptides are then recognized by the host T cells as "non-self" and initiate the acute phase of GVHD.

These results suggest that GVHD may be the net result of a combination of immune reactions.[68] Modifying any one of these responses may lead to enhancement, decrease or no effect on GVHD. An example of this has been found with T-cell depletion followed by bone marrow transplantation. The results with T-cell depletion suggest that there is a donor anti-recipient response which leads to GVHD and a recipient anti-donor response which may lead to graft failure. In the donor anti-recipient response there is also a graft-versus-leukemia effect. Evidence for a host component to GVHD is inferred from data that pretransplant TNF-α levels of the host correlated with GVHD.[69] Other evidence that the host may play an important part in GVHD is demonstrated in recipients with low NK cell reactivity had less GVHD.[70] Syngeneic T-cell-depleted bone marrow cells can lead to mixed chimerism and "prevent" GVHD (See chapter 5).[71]

## REFERENCES

1. Simpson E, Tomonari K, Lovering E. Minor transplantation antigens: Their role in shaping the T-cell repertoire. Immunol Lett 1989; 21: 39.
2. Johnson L. At how many histocompatibility loci do congenic mouse strains differ? Probability estimates and some implications. J Hered 1981; 72: 27.
3. Bailey D. How pure are inbred strains of mice? Immunol Today 1982; 3: 210.
4. Loveland B. Simpson E. The non-MHC transplantation antigens: Neither weak nor minor. Immunol Today 1986; 7: 223.
5. Roopenian D, Davis AP. Responses against antigens encoded by the H-3 histocompatibility locus: antigens stimualting class I MHC-and class II-MHC restricted T cells are encoded by separate genes. Immunogenetics 1989; 30: 335.
6. Roopenian D. What are minor histocompatibility loci? A new look at an old question. Immunol Today 1992; 13: 7.
7. Graft R, Brown DH. Estimates of histocompatibility differences between inbred mouse strains. Immunogenetics 1978; 7: 367
8. Bailey D. Hereditable histocompatibility changes: Lysogeny in mice? Transplantation 1966; 4: 482.
9. Zinkernagel R, Doherty PC. MHC-restricted cytotoxic T cells: Studies on the biological role of polymorphic major transplantation antigens determining T-cell restriction specificity, function and responsiveness. Adv Immunol 1979; 27: 52.
10. Claverie J, Kourilsky P, Langlade-Demoyden P et al. T-immunogenic peptides are constituted of rare sequence patterns. Use in the identification of T-epitopes in the human immunodeficiency virus gag protein. Eur J Immunol 1988; 18: 1547.
11. Maryanski J, Abastado JP, Kourilsky P. Specificity of peptide presentation by a set of hybrid mouse class I MHC molecules. Nature 1987; 324: 578.
12. Maryanski J, Abastado JP, McDonald RH, Kourilsky P. Intradomain $K^dD^d$ recombinants define the same regions as crucial for recognition by alloreactive or major histocompatibility complex-restricted cytolytic T cells. Eur J Immunol 1989 19: 1989.
13. Abastado J, Darche S, Godeau F, Cami B, Kourilsky P. Intramolecular recombination between partially homologous sequences in E. coli and Xenopus laevis oocytes. Proc Natl Acad Sci USA 1987; 84: 6496.

14. Abastado J, Jaulin C, Schultze MP et al. Fine mapping of epitopes in intradomain $K^d/D^d$ recombinants. J Exp Med 1987; 16: 327.

15. Healy F, Sire J, Gomard E, Yssel H, Jordan B, Levy JP. A study of functionally active amino acids involved in the interaction of HLA-A2 or HLA-A3 molecules with cytologic T lymphocytes. J Immunol 1988; 141: 2487.

16. Babbitt B, Allen PM, Matsueda G, Haber E, Unanue ER. Binding of immunogenic peptides to Ia histocompatibility molecules. Nature 1985; 317: 359.

17. Babbitt B, Matsueda G, Haber E, Unanue ER, Allen PM. Antigenic competition at the level of peptide-Ia binding. Proc Natl Acad Sci USA 1986; 83: 4509.

18. Buus S, Colon S, Smith C, Freed JH, Miles C, Grey HM. Interaction between a "processed" ovalbumin peptide and Ia molecules. Proc Natl Acad Sci USA 1986; 83: 3968.

19. Buus S, Sette A, Colon S, Jenis DM, Grey HM. Isolation and characterization of antigen-Ia complexes involved in T-cell recognition. Cell 1986; 47: 1071.

20. Watts T, McConnell HM. High-affinity flourescence peptide binding to I-$A^d$ in lipid membranes. Proc Natl Acad Sci USA 1986; 83: 9660.

21. Guillet J, Lai MZ, Briner TJ et al. Immunological self, nonself discrimination. Science 1987; 235: 865.

22. Lakey E, Casten LA, Niebling WL, Margoliash E, Pierce SK. Time dependence of B cell processing and presentation of peptide and native protein antigens. J Immunol 1988; 140: 3309.

23. Rock K, Benacerraf B. Inhibition of antigen-specific T lymphocyte activation by structurally related Ir gene-controlled polymers. Evidence of specific competition for accessory cell antigen presentation. J Exp Med 1983. 157: p. 1618.

24. Guillet J, Lai MZ, Briner TJ, Smith JA, Gefter ML. Interaction of peptide antigens and class II major histocompatibility complex antigens. Nature 1986; 324: 260.

25. Buus S, Sette A, Colon SM, Jenis DM, Grey HM. The relation between major histocompatability complex (MHC) restriction and the capacity of Ia to bind immunogenic peptides. Science 1987; 235: 1353.

26. Allen P. Antigen processing at the molecular level. Immunol Today 1987; 8: 270.

27. Fox BS, Chen C, Fraga E, Frech CA, Singh B, Schwartz RH. Functionally distinct agretopic and epitopic sites. Analysis of the dominant T-cell determinant of moth and pigeon cytochrome c with the use of synthetic peptide antigens. J Immunol 1987; 139: 1578.

28. Carbone F, Fox BS, Schwartz RH, Paterson Y. The use of hydrophobic α helix-defined peptides in delineating the T-cell determinant for pigeon cytochrome c. J Immunol 1987; 138: 1838.

29. Schwartz R. Immune response (Ir) genes of the murine major histocompatibility complex. Adv Immunol 1986; 38: 31.

30. Bastin J, Rothbard J, Davey J, Jones I, Townsend A. Use of synthetic peptides of influenza nucleoprotein to define epitopes recognized by class I-restricted cytotoxic T lymphocytes. J Exp Med 1987; 165: 1508.

31. Townsend A, Rothbard J, Gotch FM, Bahadur G, Wraith D, McMichael AJ. The epitopes of influenza nucleoprotein recognized by cytotoxic T lymphocytes can be defined with short synthetic peptides. Cell 1986; 44: 959.

32. Bjorkman P, Saper MA, Samraoui B et al. Structure of human class I histocompatibility antigen, HLA-A2. Nature 1987; 329: 506.

33. Rothbard J, Taylor WR. A sequence pattern common to T-cell epitopes. EMBO J 1988; 7: 93.

34. Brown J, Jardetzky TS, Gorga JC et al. Three-dimensional structure of the human class II histocompatibility antigen HLA-DR1. Nature 1993; 364: 33.

35. Winchester G, Sunshine GH, Nardi N, Mitchison NA. Antigen-presenting cells do not discriminate between self and nonself. Immunogenetics 1984; 19: 487.

36. Wekerle H, Schwab M, Linington C, Meyermann R. Antigen presentation in the peripheral nervous system: Schwann cells present endogenous myelin autoantigens to lymphocytes. Eur J Immunol 1986; 16: 1551.

37. Adorini L, Sette A, Buus S et al. Interaction of an immunodominant epitope with Ia molecules in T-cell activation. Proc Natl Acad Sci USA 1988; 85: 5181.

38. Adorini L, Muller S, Cardenaux F, Lehmann PV, Falcioni F and Nagy ZA. In vivo competition between self peptides and foreign antigens in T-cell activation. Nature 1988; 334.

39. Lorenz R, Allen PM. Direct evidence for functional self protein/Ia complexes in vivo. Proc Natl Acad Sci USA 1988; 85: 5220.

40. Bikoff E, Yu H, Eckhardt LA. T-cell recognition of endogenous $IgG_{2a}$ expressed in B lymphoma cells. Eur J Immunol 1988; 18: 341.

41. Jorgensen G, Hannestad K. Helper T-cell recognition of the variable domains of a mouse myeloma protein (315). Effect of the major histocompatibility complex and domain conformation. J Exp Med 1982; 155: 1587.

42. Weiss S, Bogen B. B-lymphoma cells process and present their endogenous immunoglobulin to MHC-restricted T cells. Proc Natl Acad Sci USA 1989; 86: 282.

43. Song E, Linsk R, Olson CA, McMillanM, Goodenow RS. Allogeneic cytotoxic T lymphocytes recognize an H-2 peptide in the context of a murine major histocompatibility complex class I molecule. Proc Natl Acad Sci USA 1988; 85: 1927.

44. Rammensee H, Bevan MJ. Evidence from in vitro studies that tolerance to self-antigens is MHC-restricted. Nature 1984; 308: 741.

45. Matzinger P, Zamoyska R, Waldmann H. Self tolerance is H-2 restricted. Nature 1984; 308: 738.

46. Rudensky AY, Preston-Hurlburt P, Hong S-C, Barlow A, Janeway CA. Sequence analysis of peptides bound to MHC class II molecules. Nature 1991; 353: 622.

47. Hunt D, Michel H, Dickinson TA et al. Peptides presented to the immune system by murine class II MHC molecule, I-A$^d$. Science 1992; 256: 1817.

48. Loveland B, Wang CR, Yonekawa H, Hermel E, Lindahl KF. Maternally transmitted histocompatibility antigen of mice: A hydrophobic peptide of a mitochondrially encoded protein. J Immunogenet 1990; 17: 29.

49. Brorson K, Richards S, Hunt SW. Cheroutre H, Lindahl KF, Hood L. Analysis of a new class I gene mapping to the Hmt region of the mouse. Immunogenetics 1989; 8: 3749.

50. Richards S, Bucan M, Brorson K et al. Genetic and molecular mapping of the Hmt region of mouse. EMBO J 1989; 8: 3749.

51. Speiser D, Zurcher T, Ramseier H et al. Nuclear myxovirus-resistance protein Mx is a minor histocompatibility antigen. Proc Natl Acad Sci, USA 1990; 87: 2021.

52. Wraith D, Smilek DE, Mitchell DJ, Steinman L, McDevitt HO. Antigen recognition in autoimmune encephalomyelitis and the potential for peptide-mediated immunotherapy. Cell 1989; 59: 247.

53. Adelman N, Watling DL, McDevitt HO. Treatment of (NZB x NZW) $F_1$ disease with anti-I-A monoclonal antibodies. J Exp Med 1983; 158: 1350.

54. Brostoff S, Mason DW. Experimental allergic encephalomyelitis: Successful treatment in vivo with a monoclonal antibody that recognizes T helper cells. J Immunol 1984; 133: 1938.

55. Waldor K, Hardy R, Hayakawa K, Steinman L, Herzenberg LA, Herzenberg LA. Disappearance and reappearance of B cells after in vivo treatment with monoclonal anti-I-A antibodies. Proc Natl Acad Sci (USA) 1984; 81: 2855.

56. Owhashi M, Heber-Katz E. Protection from experimental allergic encephalomyelitis conferred by a monoclonal antibody directed against a shared idiotype on rat T-cell receptors specific for myelin basic protein. J Exp Med 1988; 168: 2153.

57. Acha-Orbea H, Mitchell DJ, Timmerman L et al. Limited heterogeneity of T-cell receptors from lymphocytes mediating autoimmune encephalomyelitis allows specific immune intervention. Cell 1988; 54: 263.

58. Lamont A, Sette A, Fujinami R, Colon SM, Miles C, Grey HM. Inhibition of experimental autoimmune encephalomyelitis induction in SJL/J mice by using a peptide with high affinity for I-A$^s$ molecules. J Immunol 1990; 145: 1687.

59. Lamont A, Powell MF, Colon SM, Miles C, Grey HM, Sette A. The use of peptide analogues with improved stability and MHC binding capacity to inhibit antigen presentation in vitro and in vivo. J Immunol 1990; 144: 2493.

60. van Els C, Zantvoort E, Jacobs N, Bakker A, van Rood JJ, Goulmy E. Graft-versus-host disease associated T helper cell responses specific for minor histocompatibility antigens are mainly restricted by HLA-DR molecules. Bone Marrow Transpl 1990; 5: 365.

61. Sviland L, Pearson ADJ, Green MA et al. Expression of MHC class I and class II antigens by keratinocytes and enterocytes in acute graft-versus-host disease. Bone Marrow Transplant 1989; 4: 233

62. Sviland L, Pearson ADJ, Green MA et al. Class II antigen expression by keratinocytes and enterocytes is an early feature of graft-versus-host disease. Transplantation 1988; 46: 402.

63. Volc-Platzer B, Majdic O, Knapp W et al. Evidence of HLA-DR antigen biosynthesis by human keratinocytes in disease. J Exp Med 1984; 159: 1784.

64. Sale G, Alavaikko M, Schaefers KM, Mahan CT. Abnormal CD4:CD8 ratios and delayed germinal center reconstitution in lymph nodes of human graft recipients with graft-versus-host disease (GVHD): An immunohistological study. Exp Hematol 1992; 20: 1017.

65. Musliwietz J, Thierfelder S, Hoffmann-Fezer G, Kummer U. Antilymphocytic antibodies and bone marrow transplantation. Transplantation 1990; 49: 749.

66. Fast LD. DBA/2J and DBA/2Ha lymphocytes differ in their ability to induce graft-vs-host disease. J Immunol 1989; 143: 2489.

67. Hopkins K, Vogelsang GB, Delaney NL, Gullette DL, Santos GW, Bias WB. Implication of a gene distal to HLA-A in the etiology of graft-versus-host disease. Transpl Proc 1989; 21: 2971.

68. Gale R, Horowitz MM, Butturini A, Barrett AJ, Kolb HJ. What determines who develops graft-versus-host disease: The graft or the host (or both)? Bone Marrow Transplant 1992; 10: 99.

69. Holler E, Kolb HJ, Moller A et al. Increased serum levels of tumor necrosis factor a precede major complications of bone marrow transplantation. Blood 1990; 75: 1011.

70. Lopez C, Kirkpatrick D, Sorell M, O'Reilly RJ, Ching C. Association between pretreatment natural killer cell activity and graft-versus-host disease after stem cell transplantation. Lancet 1979; ii: 1103.

71. Sykes M, Sharabi Y, Sachs DH. Achieving alloengraftment without graft-versus-host disease: Approaches using mixed allogeneic bone marrow transplantation. Bone Marrow Transpl 1988; 3: 379.

# CYTOKINES

## INTRODUCTION

Cytokines have long been implicated in the occurrence of GVHD. Tables 5.1 and 5.2 describe the different cytokines implicated in the diagnosis of GVHD. Again, much of the study on cytokines has been in murine models, either across major histocompatibility or minor histocompatibility barriers. When a MHC mismatched BMT is performed in a mouse, both CD4 and CD8 cells release cytokines such as IL-3, GM-CSF, TNF-α and interferon-γ.[1] However, CD4+ cells seem to secrete a larger quantity of cytokines compared to CD8+ cells, suggesting that CD4+ cells may be more efficient in inducing GVHD.[2,3] M-CSF also appears to be elevated in the serum of mice with graft-versus-host reaction.[3] This suggests again that once T cells are primed, a cytokine cascade is unleashed. These cytokines may subsequently activate other T cells or other cell types such as monocytes, NK cells or NK-like cells.

Cytokines may be important not only for the donor cell proliferation but also for residual host cell proliferation. Various factors, such as IL-2, IL-4, IL-6 and IL-9, can stimulate growth in an autocrine fashion. Thus, cytokines may be very important in various steps of graft-versus-host reaction leading to GVHD. Cytokines may be important in the initial stimulation of the T cells, maintenance of the T-cell stimulation, the afferent phase of GVHD and also in the efferent phase when toxicity is manifest.

A variety of cytokines may be very important in the efferent phase of GVHD in that the release of these cytokines may drive two different subpopulations of T cells. Murine and human studies show that CD4+ cells can be divided into at least two subsets.[4-6] There are predominantly two types of T helper cells, $T_h1$ and $T_h2$ cells. This difference is based on the cytokines that these T cells produce and the cytokines to which these T cells respond (positively or negatively). $T_h1$ cells make IL-2 and interferon-γ compared to $T_h2$ cells, which make IL-4, IL-6 and IL-10. It is possible that different subpopulations of helper T cells are involved in GVHD. $T_h1$ cells make and use IL-2 for their growth. $T_h2$ cells produce IL-4 and require IL-1 or IL-4 for proliferation. Production and release of these cytokines may influence which subsets of the CD4 cells predominate in GVHD. A predominance of $T_h1$ cells could lead to activation of CTLs and subsequent GVHD, compared to a preponderance of $T_h2$ cells leading to a humoral response and prevention of GVHD.

### Table 5.1. Single cytokines implicated in GVHD

| Cytokine | Observation | Reference |
|---|---|---|
| INF-β | • Increased INF-β in mice with GVHD | 28 |
| INF-γ | • Antibodies against INF-γ prevented intestinal pathology in a murine model of GVHD<br>• Increased circulating levels of INF-γ in humans following BMT in patients with GVHD | 29 |
| TNF | • Polyclonal antibodies against TNF prevented GVHD in adult and newborn murine models<br>• Increased levels in patients with GVHD or prior to other catastrophic events (e.g. sepsis)<br>• Increased mRNA levels of TNF in rats with GVHD | 24-26 |
| IL-1 | • IL-1 receptor antagonist prevents GVHD morbidity and mortality | 17 |
| IL-2 | • IL-2 increased mortality in class I, but not class II incompatible GVHD in mice and rats<br>• IL-2 increased mortality following BMT across minor histocompatibility antigens<br>• Anti-IL-2 antibodies blocked GVHD in a murine model<br>• Monoclonal antibodies against IL-2 have been used to treat patients with GVHD with encouraging results<br>• IL-2 given early following T-depleted bone marrow graft prevents GVHD, if given late it accelerates GVHD | 11-16 |

Adapted with permission from Jadus & Wepsic (ref. 38)

### Table 5.2 Combination cytokines implicated in GVHD

| Combination Cytokines | Observation | Reference |
|---|---|---|
| IL-3/GM-CSF | • T cells of mice with GVHD spontaneously produce IL-3 and GM-CSF | 34 |
| IL-4/IL-1 | • Enhanced GVHD mortality in mice given IL-4 and IL-1 | 35 |
| IL-4/IL-5 | • Enhanced production of autoantibodies in mice with chronic GVHD | 36 |
| M-CSF/CSF1 | • Increased levels in mice with GVHD | 37 |
| IL-2, IL-3, IL-4, CSF | • Produced by T cells when minor or MHC differences are found following BMT | 18 |
| IL-2, IL-3, IL-6, TNF, IFN | • Produced by CD4[+] clones in animals with GVHD. T-cell clones producing TNF-α can transfer lethal GVHD | 8, 18 |
| IL-1, IL-6, TNF, IFN | • Expressed by Con A or LPS in splenocytes of mice undergoing GVHD | 19 |

Adapted with permission from Jadus & Wepsic (ref. 38)

Cytokines are also important in other minor abnormalities seen in GVHD. For example, TNF-α and interferon-γ and TGF-β could inhibit differentiation and marrow reconstitution.[7,8] Other cytokines may lead to bone marrow fibrosis or changes in the stromal microenvironment.[9] Several of these factors may drive stem cells towards differentiation ("stem cell steal") and lead to depletion of these progenitor cells.

## INTERLEUKINS

One of the most studied interleukins is IL-2. IL-2 added exogenously during the first week of graft-versus-host reaction enhances the severity and mortality associated with class I MHC disparate transplantation. In contrast, IL-2 does not cause a similar increase in class II disparate BMT.[10] This has also been observed in a rat model of GVHD.[11] In addition, there was an increase in relative numbers of large granular lymphocytes, as well as NK and LAK activity which could be further augmented by incubation with IL-2. IL-2 increased the expression of interferon-γ in GVHD cells. However, this does not appear to be true in a murine model of minor histocompatibility differences.[12] The role of IL-2 is even more complicated in that high doses of IL-2 seem to prevent GVHD induced by allogeneic T cells when given in conjunction with syngeneic T-cell depleted bone marrow (see below).[13,14] High doses of IL-2 administered over a short period beginning on the day of bone marrow transplantation mediate a protective effect against GVHD in mice while preserving the ability to treat alloengraftment. This protective effect is augmented by administration of T-cell depleted syngeneic marrow and appears to be dependent upon the early use of IL-2. There does not seem to be a decrease in the graft-versus-leukemia effect. The mechanism of protection by IL-2 administration might involve the in vivo activation of natural killer and/or LAK cells. To evaluate this hypothesis, the effect of IL-2 administration on the number of NK cells or NK-mediated cytotoxic activity in recipients of GVHD producing cells was tested. NK cells and LAK cells were depleted in vivo with monoclonal antibodies to evaluate the effect of IL-2-induced GVHD protection. The results from this study demonstrate

1.  That there is no change in the number of NK cells in the spleen of IL-2-treated compared to control recipients
2.  NK activity is not increased in IL-2-treated recipients compared to control recipients
3.  The depletion of NK and LAK precursors influence the time course of GVHD mortality in a complex fashion
4.  IL-2-induced GVHD protection is largely independent of the activity of an NK or LAK cell population of donor or host origin

This study concluded that IL-2-induced GVHD protection was primarily the activity of non-LAK-protected cell populations. Conversely, these cells may direct an inhibitory effect on the responding donor cell population as they encounter the host antigen. A follow-up study demonstrated that there are consistent delays in splenic repopulation by allogeneic cells after BMT in IL-2-treated animals compared with their untreated cohorts.[15] There was a greater reduction in donor splenic T-cell population in the first few days after BMT in IL-2-treated animals. Splenic cells with CD3+ CD4-

CD8⁻ phenotype were increased in IL-2-treated animals at days 3 and 4 after BMT. The phenotype of the cells resembles that of the bone marrow-derived cells which have been previously shown to inhibit GVHD. This is just one possible mechanism for the protective effect of IL-2. These results suggest that IL-2 treatment leads to elimination or inactivation of donor T cells. IL-2 may mediate this effect by decreasing expansion of GVH reactive donor T cells in the early period after BMT. The ability to disassociate the GVHD promoting activity of donor T cells from the capacity to promote engraftment and graft-versus-leukemia effect is an exciting prospect for the use of IL-2 clinically in allogeneic BMT.

High-dose IL-2, when begun on the day of bone marrow transplantation has a protective effect against GVHD, especially when coadministered with T-cell depleted syngeneic bone marrow cells. One possibility is that IL-2 induces lymphokine-activated killer (LAK) cells that may mediate GVHD protection. Conversely, adoptive transfer studies failed to provide evidence that the treatment of lethally irradiated mice with IL-2 activates protective host-derived or syngeneic marrow-derived cell populations that could be adoptively transferred to lethally irradiated secondary recipients receiving allogeneic bone marrow. Moreover, treatment of lethally irradiated mice with a complete 2.5 day course of IL-2 prior to administration of allogeneic cells did not lead to GVHD protection. If the addition of IL-2 was delayed for a week, then exogenous IL-2 accelerated the GVHD mortality. Recent data demonstrate that administration of high doses of IL-2 early after BMT provides marked protection against GVHD. Similarly, the graft-versus-leukemia effect of donor T cells against a leukemia/lymphoma is preserved. This is interesting because the protective ability of IL-2 against GVHD appears to be paradoxical. Perhaps LAK cells which can inhibit GVHD are activated by this course of IL-2.[14] These experiments suggest either that IL-2 directly inhibits GVHD reactivity of the donor GVH-reactive cells or that the GVH reactivity is decreased by IL-2 during the period of interaction between donor and host cell type.[16] Two other important T-cell activating cytokines include IL-1 and IL-4. An IL-1 receptor antagonist was able to prevent mortality by more than 70% in a murine BMT model.[17]

The roles of other cytokines in chronic autoimmune GVHD in a murine model have been investigated specifically in vivo administration of interferon-γ, anti-interferon-γ or anti-interleukin-4 monoclonal antibodies.[18] Early treatment with anti-IL-4 monoclonal antibody or interferon-γ decreased hypogammaglobulinemia specifically of serum IgE and IgG1 but had no effect on IgG2a. Anti-interferon-γ monoclonal antibody increased serum IgE and IgG1 while reducing IgG2a. The increase in serum immunoglobulins could be correlated with an increase in spontaneous secretion of IL-4, IL-5, IL-6 and spleen cultures from anti-interferon-γ monoclonal antibody-treated GVHD mice. Neither anti-interferon-γ monoclonal antibody or interferon-γ treatments altered the disease course. On the other hand, anti-IL-4 treatment delayed proteinuria and death in mice with GVHD. These observations suggest another important cytokine: that of IL-4 in the immune complex mediated glomerulonephritis of chronic graft-versus-host disease.

It is not surprising that cytokine synthesis is under complex and multilevel control. One level of control involves the ability of cytokines from one cell type to modulate production of other cytokines by different cell types, inducing a cytokine cascade. One such example is tumor necrosis factor's (TNF) ability to induce IL-6 synthesis. IL-6 is a pleiotropic 21-30 kd glycoprotein produced by various cell types. T-cell maturation and differentiation depends on IL-6. Moreover, IL-6 provides key signals for T-cell proliferative and cytotoxic responses. The involvement of cytokines in acute GVHD led to serial serum measurements of IL-6 in 22 allogeneic marrow recipients who developed acute GVHD.[19] This study found that elevation of serum levels IL-6 tended to precede the onset of GVHD. These data suggest that not only is TNF and interferon-γ involved GVHD, but IL-6 is likely also involved in the cytokine cascade.

Other evidence for the involvement of TNF and IL-6 has been supported by the rapid reappearance of monocytes after bone marrow transplantation.[20] Production of both of these cytokines can be induced as early as 10-14 days following BMT at the very beginning of engraftment, indicating that the regeneration of the monocyte system recovers rapidly after BMT. Depletion and neutralization experiments confirm that the monocytes are the cellular source of inducible cytokine secretion after BMT. Inducible cytokine production from monocytes was not affected by acute or chronic GVHD or by allogeneic or autologous BMT, nor by treatment with cyclosporine A. The coincident appearance of monocyte-derived cytokines and of GVHD suggests a role of these cytokines in GVHD.

## TUMOR NECROSIS FACTOR

Tumor necrosis factor-α (TNF-α) is a polypeptide (17.3 kd) and mediates a wide range of inflammatory and immune responses involving cells of epithelial and myeloid origin. TNF-α was originally discovered as a cytotoxic factor for tumor cells and as a factor involved in cachexia induced by chronic illnesses such as cancer or acquired immunodeficiency syndrome. At lower levels, TNF-α plays an important protective role in stimulating chemotaxis and antimicrobial activities of white blood cells. During chronic illness TNF-α secretion can be elevated, giving rise to cachexia, hemorrhage, necrosis and ultimately death. Moreover, keratinocytes can be induced to synthesize TNF-α.[21]

Two of the major factors implicated in GVHD have been TNF-α and interferon-γ. The interest in the role of TNF and GVHD derived from studies of the role of the gut flora in GVHD. It has been known for many years that gnotobiotic (free of pathogens) mice are protected from GVHD following BMT. Any re-colonization of a gram-negative bacteria led to the recurrence of GVHD. Clinical data support gut decontamination and laminar flow rooms which may decrease the severity of GVHD in selected patients.[22] It is likely that the damage from radiation and chemotherapy to the gut allows gut flora and endotoxins to enter the circulation. Support for this theory comes from a trial of monoclonal antibody against endotoxin that seems to protect mice against GVHD.[23] Endotoxin is a well-known stimulus for cytokine production and release, specifically of TNF. Piguet et al used a polyclonal neutralizing antibody against TNF-α to demonstrate a reduction in GVHD-associated mortality by 70%, which also diminished lesions in the skin and the intestines.[24] Similar results were obtained using a neutralizing antibody against murine TNF with reduction of splenomegaly in neonatal graft-versus-host reactions.[25] In human allogeneic BMT, four to nine times the levels of TNF were found in patients with grade II-IV GVHD compared to those with grade I or no GVHD. These elevated levels occurred prior to the onset of clinical disease.[26] Similar results were reported in 11 out of 12 patients who had elevated levels of TNF-α with acute GVHD.[19] However, elevated levels of TNF is not a universal finding since there are patients with acute GVHD who do not display elevated levels of TNF in the serum.[26] Moreover, elevated TNF levels were found in other disease states such as endothelial leakage syndrome, interstitial pneumonitis and veno-occlusive disease of the liver.

## INTERFERON

Several studies evaluated cytokine production by mice undergoing acute GVHD to determine whether there is a characteristic panel of secretions that accounts for the in vitro specific activity of GVHD spleen cells. Particular focus has been placed on the potential role of interferon-γ required for the expression of natural suppressor cells activity. Natural suppressor cells are potent nonspecific inhibitors of proliferative responses in vitro. One study demonstrated that graft-versus-host spleen cells proliferate poorly in response to Concanavalin A (Con A) and produce high levels of interferon-γ when exposed to mitogens. Proliferation of these GVHD spleen cells is substantially enhanced by the addition of anti-interferon-γ antibodies.[27] These results indicate spleen cell capacity of mice undergoing GVHD for cytokine production can be affected by the action of some of these pharmacological agents. Splenocytes of GVHD mice exhibit an increased capacity to produce IL-1, IL-6, TNF-α when stimulated by lipopolysaccharide. This enhanced capacity diminishes following in vivo treatment with immunosuppressive drugs. Conc A stimulates GVHD spleen cells producing significantly lower levels of IL-2 but higher levels of interferon-γ compared to syngeneic spleen cells. These results differ from other reports suggesting that the majority of interferon produced by Con A-stimulated spleen cells is interferon-α and β, not interferon-γ. The evidence suggests that interferon-γ mediates the immunosuppressive activity of graft-versus-host spleen cells while IL-1 may be involved in the development of splenomegaly.

Interferon can be detected in the serum of mice with GVHD.[28] Spleen cells from mice with chronic GVHD produce interferon spontaneously in vitro. Unlike normal spleen cells that produce interferon-γ, the spleen cells from mice with GVHD produce interferon-β.[29] However, in vivo studies demonstrated that interferon-γ is found in the peri-arteriolar lymphoid regions of the spleen of mice with GVHD. In contrast, interferon-β is found in a much more diffuse pattern in both lymphoid and red pulp areas. Interferon-γ is also increased in patients with GVHD. Circulating interferon-γ is four-fold higher in patients with grade II-IV acute GVHD compared to those without significant GVHD.[30] Using a monoclonal anti-interferon-γ antibody led to the reduction of the intestinal pathology in two MHC-mismatched murine models. Another murine model of minor histocompatibility antigens suggests that liver and spleen cells suppress the proliferation of mitogen-stimulated normal spleen cells in a MHC-unrestricted manner.[31] The suppressor activity from spleen cells was mediated by natural suppressor cells and involved a soluble suppressor factor. Interferon-γ and prostaglandins were shown to partially mediate the observed suppressive activity.

An important effect of selected cytokines is the ability to induce higher expression of MHC class I and class II antigens. Clearly the cells with low expression of MHC class I molecules will not be lysed by host-specific killer cells.[32] It is possible that, if leukemic cells also exhibit such features, induction or increase in the class I or II MHC molecules may render them more susceptible to cytolysis by cytotoxic T cells.

Another study demonstrated the importance of cytokines in the regulation of cellular immune responses. The study analyzed endogenous interferon-γ levels in human BMT recipients and related the finding to the conditioning regimen and clinical complications and demonstrated that both GVHD and infections strongly influence the endogenous release of interferon-γ.[33] The kinetics of interferon-γ elevation differed between BMT recipients with GVHD and infectious complications following BMT. Increasing interferon-γ levels were seen during the infection subsequent to the clinical manifestation, whereas in GVHD it preceded the disease manifestation.

## REFERENCES

1. Korngold R, Sprent J. T-cell subsets and graft-versus-host disease. Transplantation 1987; 44: 335.
2. Mason D. Subsets of T cells in the rat mediating lethal graft-versus-host disease. Transplantation 1981 32: 222.
3. Fong T, Mosmann TR. Alloreactive murine CD8+ T-cell clones secrete the Th1 pattern of cytokines. J Immunol 1990; 144: 1744.
4. Kapsenberg M, Wierenga EA, Bos JD, Jansen HM. Functional subsets of allergen-reactive human CD4+ T cells. Immunol Today 1991; 392.
5. Mosmann T, Moore KE. The role of IL10 in cross-regulation of Th1 and Th2 responses. Immunol Today 1991; 12: A49.
6. Street N, Mosmann TR. Functional diversity of T lymphocytes due to secretion of different cytokine patterns. FASEB J 1991; 5: 171.
7. Ohta M, Greenberger JS, Anklesaria R, Bassols A, Massague J. Two forms of transforming growth factor-beta distinguished by multipotential haemapoietic progenitor cells. Nature 1987; 329: 539.
8. Broxmeyer H, Williams DE, Lu L et al. The suppressive influences of human tumor necrosis factor on bone marrow hematopoietic progenitor cells from normal donors and patients with leukemia: Synergism of tumor necrosis factor and interferon-gamma. J Immunol 1986; 136: 4487.
9. Ishihara K, Shimamine T. Structural changes of the murine bone marrow in graft-versus-host reaction. Path Res Pract 1980; 169: 84.
10. Jadus M, Peck AB. Lethal murine graft-versus-host disease in the absence of detectable cytotoxic T lymphocytes. Transplantation 1983; 36: 281.
11. Clancy J, Goral J, Kovacs EJ, Ellis T. Role of recombinant interleukin-2 (rIL-2) and large granular lymphocytes (LGLs) in acute rat graft-versus-host disease (GVHD). Transpl Proc 1989; 21: 88.
12. Merluzzi V, Welte K, Last-Barney K et al. Production and response to interleukin-2 in vitro and in vivo after bone marrow transplantation in mice. J Immunol 1985; 134: 2426.

13. Sykes M, Romick ML, Hoyles KA, Sachs DH. In vivo administration of inter-leukin-2 plus T-cell depleted syngeneic marrow prevents graft-versus-host disease mortality and permits alloengraftment. J Exp Med 1990; 171: 645.

14. Sykes M, Abraham VS. The mechanism of IL-2-mediated protection against GVHD in mice,. Transplantation 1992; 53: 1063.

15. Abraham V, Sachs DH, Sykes M. Mechanism of protection from graft-versus-host disease mortality by IL-2. J Immunol 1992; 148: 3746.

16. Abraham V, Sykes M. Mechanism of the anti-GVHD effect IL-2: I. Protective host-type cell populations are not induced by IL-2 treatment alone. Bone Marrow Transpl 1991; 7 Suppl: 29.

17. McCarthy P, Abhyankar S, Neben S et al. Inhibition of interleukin-1 receptor antagonist prevents graft-versus-host disease. Blood 1991; 78: 1915.

18. Umland S, Razac S, Nahrebne DK, Seymour BW. Effects of in vivo administration of interferon (IFN)-γ, anti-IFN-γ, or anti-interleukin-4 monoclonal antibodies in chronic autoimmune graft-versus-host disease. Clin Immunol Immunopathol 1992; 63: 66.

19. Symington F, Symington BE, Liu PY, Viguet H, Santhanam U, Sehgal PB. The relationship of serum IL-6 levels to acute graft-versus-host disease and hepatorenal disease after human bone marrow transplantation. Transplantation 1992; 54: 457.

20. Pechumer H, Leinisch E, Bender-Gotze C, Ziegler-Heitmrock L. Recovery of monocytes after bone marrow transplantation-rapid reappearance of tumor necrosis factor alpha and interleukin-6 production. Transplantation 1991; 52: 698.

21. Cheng J, Turksen K, Yu QC, Shreiber H, Teng M, Fuchs EM. Cachexia and graft-vs-host-disease-type skin changes in keratin promoter-driven TNF-α transgenic mice. Genes & Devel 1992; 6: 1444.

22. Storb R, Prentice RL, Buckner CD et al. Graft-versus-host disease and survival in patients with aplastic anemia treated by marrow grafts from HLA-identical siblings. Beneficial effect of a protective enviroment. N Engl J Med 1983; 308: 302.

23. Moore R, Lampert IA, Chia Y, Aber VR, Cohen J. Effect of immunization with Escherichia coli J5 in graft-versus-host disease induced by minor histocompatibility antigens in mice. Transplantation 1987; 44: 249.

24. Piguet P, Grau GE, Allet B, Vassalli P. Tumor necrosis factor/cachectin is an effector of skin and gut lesions of the acute phase of graft-vs-host disease. J Exp Med 1987; 166: 1280.

25. Shalaby M, Fendly B, Sheehan K, Schreiber RD, Ammann AJ. Prevention of the graft-versus-host reaction in newborn mice by antibodies to tumor necrosis factor-alpha. Transplantation 1989; 47: 1057.

26. Holler E, Kolb HJ, Moller A et al. Increased serum levels of tumor necrosis factor α precede major complications of bone marrow transplantation. Blood 1990; 75: 1011.

27. Smith S, Terminelli C, Kenworthy PD, Bott L. A study of cytokine production in acute graft-vs-host disease. Cell Immunol 1991; 134: 336.

28. Reyes V, Klimpel GR. Interferon α/β synthesis during acute graft-versus-host disease. Transplantation 1987; 43: 412.

29. Cleveland M, Annable CR, Klimpel GR. In vivo and in vitro production of IFN-β and IFN-γ during graft vs host disease. J Immunol 1988; 141: 3349.

30. Mowat A. Antibodies to IFN-γ prevent immunologically mediated intestinal damage in murine graft-versus-host reaction. Immunology 1989; 68: 18.

31. Howell C, Yoder TY, Vierling JM. Suppressor function of liver mononuclear cells isolated during murine chronic graft-vs-host disease. Cell Immunol 1992; 140: 54.

32. Huber C, Niederwieser D. Role of cytokines and major histocompatibilty complex antigens in graft-versus-host disease: In vitro studies using T-cell lines and keratinocytes or hemopoietic targets. Haematol Blood Transf 1990; 33: 652.

33. Niederwieser D, Herold M, Woloszczuk W et al. Endogenous IFN-gamma during human bone marrow transplantation. Transplantation 1990; 50: 620.

34. Hakim F, Pluznik DH, Shearer GM. Factors contributing to the decrease in concanavalin A induced colony stimulating factors in acute suppressive graft-versus-host disorder. Transplantation 1990; 49: 781.

35. Atkinson K, Matias C, Guiffre A et al. In vivo administration of granulocyte colony stimulating factor (G-CSF), granulocyte-macrophage CSF, interleukin-1 (IL1) and IL-4; alone and in combination after allogeneic murine hematopoietic stem cell transplantation. Blood 1991; 77:1376.

36. Dobashi K, Ono S, Murakami S, Takahama T, Katoh Y, Hamaoka T. Polyclonal B cell activation by a B cell differentiation factor, B151-TRF2. J Immunol 1987; 143:15.

37. Proloran V, Raventos-Suarez C, Bartocci A, Lucas J, Stanley ER, Gibbons JJ. Alterations in the expression of colony stimulating factor-1 and its receptor during an acute graft-versus-host reaction in mice. J Immunol 1990; 145:3256.

38. Jadus MR, Vepsic HT. The role of cytokines in graft-versus-host reactions and disease. Bone Marrow Transplant 1992; 10:1.

# CHAPTER 6

# TOLERANCE

## INTRODUCTION

One of the most impressive outcomes of allogeneic bone marrow transplantation is the development of tolerance. This is a state of mutual existence between the host and the graft, devoid of obvious medical complications. Unlike solid organ transplantation, patients who receive allogeneic bone marrow may have all the immunosuppressants stopped if no GVHD develops after an appropriate course of immunosuppressants. The patient remains well with a normal, functioning hematopoietic system. Therefore, in this state, the graft is tolerant of the host and the host is tolerant of the graft (in cases of mixed chimerism). When this state does not develop, GVHD occurs or the graft is rejected (host-versus-graft). Understanding tolerance is critical in understanding and developing safer methods for allogeneic transplantation. If we could always induce tolerance in the graft-versus-host direction, then GVHD would be prevented. Tolerance in the host-versus-graft direction is achieved with more effective elimination of the residual host lymphocytes which are responsible for graft rejection. Finally, the induction tolerance in the graft-versus-host direction would also allow the engraftment of allogeneic solid organs without the need of chronic life-long immunosuppression. Clinical evidence shows that BMT results in specific tolerance to organ transplantation, when the donor of the bone marrow is also the donor of the solid organ.[1] This has been specifically shown for patients who receive a renal transplant following bone marrow transplantation. Various methods thought to be important in tolerance are listed in Table 6.1.

---

**Table 6.1. Methods implicated in the establishment of tolerance**

- Clonal deletion
- Clonal anergy
- Active suppression
    veto cells
    suppressor cells
- Lack of costimulatory signal

---

The ability of cells from unresponsive animals to respond to donor-specific alloantigens in in vivo and in vitro experiments suggests that alloreactive cells are present in these tolerant animals but are prevented from effecting rejection. This is in contrast to the main mechanism of maintaining graft survival, the occurrence of clonal deletion. It is important in clinical transplantation that tolerance to a graft can occur without clonal deletion. The mechanisms responsible for the establishment of tolerance after BMT are likely to be complex and not yet completely understood. The main factors involved in the establishment (or lack) of tolerance are

1. extent of the disparity of HLA matching[2,3]
2. susceptibility of different targets of cytotoxic effector cells[4,5]
3. differences in specific lymphokine levels[6-8]
4. type of immunosuppressive therapy[3,9]
5. clonal effects on donor or host-specific precursor cytotoxic T lymphocytes[10-12]
6. various suppressor cell mechanisms[10,13,14]

However, the four major mechanisms involved for the induction or maintenance of tolerance to alloantigens are (1) clonal deletion, (2) clonal anergy, (3) active suppression and (4) lack of costimulatory signal.

## CLONAL DELETION

Clonal deletion refers to the specific elimination of unique cells which recognize allogeneic antigens through their specific receptors. Thus, all cells which recognize either self- or alloantigens can be removed by this mechanism. This method of tolerance comes from a study in mice that eliminated a unique type of T-cell receptors which carry a specific Vβ chain.[15,16] These Vβ chains can directly recognize antigens called superantigens. This recognition is unique in that it does not require the full αβ component of the T-cell receptor. Mice that are known to carry these unique superantigens do not have any T cells which express the specific Vβ to recognize these superantigens. These T cells are deleted and the gene product is not found. Therefore, if the unique Vβ chains that recognize these superantigens, e.g., the minor lymphocyte stimulatory locus (MLS) antigens, are found, mice that carry this unique Vβ will not express these superantigens because an autoimmune disease would occur. Thus, these T cells which carry this unique Vβ can recognize these superantigens.

A second piece of data to support clonal deletion comes from transgenic mice carrying a T-cell receptor specific for self-class I MHC-restricted peptide or a class I-restricted antigen.[17,18] When these mice were analyzed, there was a marked depletion of CD8+ T cells bearing that self-reactive T-cell receptor. This suggests that there is a similar mechanism of clonal deletion for developing T cells which recognize self-determinants that can act as conventional transplantation antigens. These T cells are then destroyed. The site where this occurs is the thymus. Any T cell which carries a stronger activity against these self-antigens presented on the thymus is therefore eliminated.[19]

## ANERGY

Anergy has also been explored. This is a phenomena that is the opposite of what one would expect to occur with T cells when the T-cell receptor is engaged. In certain circumstances, rather than increasing the T cell responses to this particular antigen, engagement of the antigen with the T-cell receptor leads to a state of unresponsiveness. In vitro evidence suggests that certain antigens can render these T cells unresponsive when a costimulatory signal is not delivered by the antigen-presenting cell.[20] Probably the best known mechanism is the B7/CD28 costimulatory signal.[21,22] This T-cell anergy can occur either centrally, such as in the thymus, or peripherally, in the circulation. Under certain circumstances, these anergic T cells can become activated.

## ACTIVE SUPPRESSION

### SUPPRESSOR T CELLS/NATURAL SUPPRESSOR CELLS

Active suppression of T cells can also occur. These are the so-called suppressor cells initially described by Richard Gershon.[23] These cells have been implicated in the maintenance of self- and allotolerance. The functional evidence of specific suppression has been demonstrated and can be transplanted; however, it has been difficult to clone some of these specific cells.[24-27] An example of specific suppressor cells comes from different subsets of T cells in adult mouse bone marrow and spleen which can induce or suppress acute GVHD.[28] Fractionation of normal adult mouse spleen and bone marrow cells performed by discontinuous percoll density gradients can demonstrate this phenomenon. Fractionated low density cells (1.050-1.060 g/ml) completely suppressed acute lethal GVHD when coinjected with unfractionated spleen cells into sublethally irradiated allogeneic mice. On the other hand, high-density (1.075-1.090 g/ml) spleen fractions induced acute GVHD in these allogeneic recipients. This phenomena is not observed using bone marrow cells. This low density fraction of both bone marrow and spleen cells had a marked depletion of typical $\alpha\beta$ CD4$^+$ or CD8$^+$ T cells and a rather predominant population of $\alpha\beta$ CD4$^-$ CD8$^-$ T cells. A purified population of these CD4$^-$ and CD8$^-$ T cells suppressed GVHD.[28] Similar cells have also been observed using wheat germ agglutination in both mice and monkeys. Moreover, these fractions appear to be enriched for hematopoietic precursor cells.[29,30] These cells are the so-called natural suppressor cells. Although these cells resemble NK cells morphologically, they do not express NK cell surface markers.[31]

Natural suppressor cells are capable of suppressing immunological responses in a nonspecific manner. Natural suppressor cells are found in the spleen of mice undergoing chronic GVHD. These natural suppressor cells appear to be dependent upon lymphokines for the ability to manifest the suppression. Interferon-$\gamma$ is necessary for natural suppressor activity as shown by using anti-interferon-$\gamma$ antibody. Anti-interferon-$\gamma$ antibody was able to remove the ability of natural suppressor cells to suppress proliferation. Moreover, the anti-interferon-$\gamma$ antibody removes the ability of IL-2 to enhance natural suppressor cell suppression of Concanavalin A responses.[32]

### VETO CELLS

The inhibitory activity of bone marrow cells resembles a veto cell phenomenon in that the bone marrow cells can suppress anti-self-response.[33] Bone marrow cells abrogate adoptively transferred second set rejections and thus share with the graft the antigen recognized by the sensitized cells. Veto cells are not required to recognize the cells that they inactivate. When a T cell recognizes an antigen on the surface of the veto cell, the T cell becomes inactivated. This is a unidirectional recognition leading to suppression of an anti-self-response, thus defining characteristics of veto cells. Veto cell activity has been found in tissues rich in immature T cells such as the bone marrow, thymus, fetal liver and spleen and among cultured adult spleen cells.[34] Veto cells are able to suppress specifically the cytotoxic immune response against target cells syngeneic to themselves without inhibition to the immune response against unrelated target cells. Although the role of veto cells in the establishment of natural tolerance to self is unknown, the development of unresponsiveness to allografts has been attributed in part to veto cells.

Veto cells are also important in downregulating allogeneic responses. Veto cells inactivate T cells recognizing antigens expressed on the veto cells. This results in unique suppression affecting only those T cells responding to these antigens. Veto cells have been implicated in the induction of graft-versus-host tolerance in the setting of marrow engraftment.[35,36] These veto cells may also be important in donor-specific transfusion suppression that is observed following solid organ transplantation.[35] There is a unique state of hypo-responsiveness which is induced following blood transfusion, e.g., renal graft recipients with improvement in graft survival. No clinical data suggest that a similar form of immunosuppression occurs following BMT in humans. Actually, the opposite appears to be true. Patients with aplastic anemia who receive multiple blood transfusions appear to become sensitized to the alloantigens and have less favorable outcomes. This is not surprising, however, since the induction of tolerance should be in the donor and not the recipient (for prevention of GVHD). There is a murine model where pretreatment of prospective donors of hematopoietic cells with a single recipient-specific blood transfusion can significantly decrease the morbidity and mortality of GVHD.[37] This beneficial effect could be demonstrated for MHC class II, but not class I, differences. The suppressive effect was proportional to the amount of recipient strain blood used for transfusion, and repeated transfusions were not more effective than a single one. The time between the transfusion and transplantation was important, with the best interval being four days. This beneficial effect was specific since third party transfusions did not affect GVHD. The improvement in GVHD was due to suppression of anti-host response. Another study demonstrated the effect of donor bone marrow on second set graft rejection responses initiated by sensitized spleen cells. It showed that donor bone marrow cells abrogate the cytotoxic effects of alloreactive sensitized spleen cells.[33] The authors suggest that there may be veto cells in the donor bone marrow that may specifically abrogate the secondary response.

Veto cell-mediated suppression of CTL responses has been proposed as one mechanism by which self-tolerance is maintained. Cyclosporine-inhibited veto cell-mediated suppression of CTL responses.[38] This inhibition correlated with the lack of clonal deletion of CTL precursors by veto cells in the presence of cyclosporine. Cyclosporine also exerts effects through cytotoxic T-lymphocyte precursors and not through veto cells, indicating that CTL precursors may play an active role in their own deletion by veto cells.

# MIXED CHIMERISM

Bone marrow chimeras and tolerance can be achieved in otherwise normal adult animals. Much of this work has been carried out by Sykes and Sachs. They have demonstrated in a murine model that, when T-cell depleted allogeneic and T cell-depleted syngeneic bone marrow is coadministered, mixed chimerism occurs.[35,39-42] When mixed chimerism occurs, there is protection from GVHD and specific tolerance induced to donor antigens. These experiments using allogeneic bone marrow coadministered with T-cell depleted syngeneic marrow suggests that, for such grafting mechanisms, the addition of unmanipulated host syngeneic cells is important to confer immune responsiveness to the host following transplantation. The persistence of host type lymphoid hematopoietic cells is likely to provide continued deletion of host-reactive T-cell clones.[43] Murine experiments suggest that clonal deletion is likely to be the predominant mechanism in host-versus-graft tolerance following allogeneic transplantation. Suppressor cells appear not to be involved in the maintenance of tolerance. Tolerance can be broken readily in such chimeras by administering a relatively small number of nontolerant recipient type spleen cells.[42]

Another possible method to achieve mixed chimerism is by a vascularized bone marrow graft.[44] This unique method of grafting uses composite tissue (a femur) which contains many tissues such as skin, muscle, nerve, blood vessels, bone and bone marrow. When such grafts are transplanted into unmodified hosts, mixed chimerism without GVHD is established. No immunologic or radiological immunosuppression is needed. These results suggest that low-level, stable, mixed chimerism may be very important in tolerance induction.

It may be possible experimentally to induce tolerance utilizing genetic engineering. One such approach is to transfer donor type MHC genes into bone marrow hematopoietic stem cells. Reconstituted recipients with autologous bone marrow expressing an allogeneic class I gene appear to confer tolerance to the product of that gene. Studies are in progress to attempt to use a similar approach of induced tolerance across a class II barrier in an animal model. Allogeneic thymus transplantation may be another means to induce transplantation tolerance. Ninety percent of mice who received total lymphoid irradiation and allogeneic thymus grafts permanently accepted allogeneic bone marrow grafts. These mice are specifically tolerant to this allogeneic MHC antigen.[45] Such an approach would be an interesting method to study T-cell maturation in an allogeneic environment, while inducing specific alloantigen tolerance. Although the ability of these cells to induce donor-specific tolerance across MHC barriers has been recognized for many years, as well as the description of neonatally induced tolerance, it is now clear that this tolerance can be broken by a large number of naive host-type lymphocytes. The ability to break tolerance was initially ascribed to the restoration of clones which were eliminated during the induction of tolerance.[46-48] More specifically, this ability to break tolerance seems to be related to CD4+ T cells but not CD8+ T cells in a mixed allogeneic chimera.[49] This was surprising in that CD8+ cells appear to be the primary effectors in mediating the resistance to alloengraftment and mixed allogeneic reconstitution. Again, it may be that specific cytokines produced by the CD4+ T cells are the driving force behind the loss of chimerism intolerance.

## TOLERANCE TO MINOR HISTOCOMPATIBILITY ANTIGENS

Much of the difficulty in analyzing most of the published data on T-cell tolerance is that data gathered under certain experimental conditions may not apply to others. That is, results from studies of self-tolerance or tolerance across MHC differences may not be directly extrapolated to mechanisms found for minor histocompatibility differences. Other variables such as the status of the thymus and developmental stage of the T cell may have a direct effect on the development of tolerance. Following tissue transplantation, blood transfusion or BMT, donor antigens are presented to the host's mature T cells. In this case, tolerance is probably secondary to peripheral mechanisms such as clonal anergy or suppression. The available data suggest that suppressor cells are both necessary and sufficient to maintain graft-versus-host tolerance.[50] The development of tolerance in BMT, however, is more complex since both donor mature T cells and immature thymocytes encounter all the host antigens at a time when host antigen-presenting cells are depleted and donor antigen-presenting cells are just emerging. In this setting, a murine model for BMT across minor histocompatibility differences suggests that (1) host and donor APCs can present antigen to donor T cells; (2) the number of alloreactive donor T cells will determine if GVHD will or will not occur and (3) GVHD can be triggered only by a limited number of dominant minor histocompatibility antigens. Moreover, in this experimental model, there was no evidence for natural suppressor cells, veto cells or anti-idiotypic suppressor cells.[51]

## LACK OF COSTIMULATORY SIGNAL

As mentioned previously, the donor-derived T cells and possibly NK or NK-like cells are important in GVHD. Engrafted T cells recognize the host minor histocompatibility antigens (in matched related donor transplants) in the context of either class I or class II MHC molecules. The first signal is when the T-cell receptor recognizes the peptide fragment, the minor histocompatibility antigen, which is bound to the MHC class I or class II antigen. The second signal, or so-called costimulus, is provided by a different receptor ligand interaction. This second signal occurs when either the CD4 or the CD8 molecule binds to the invariant determinants in the class II or the class I MHC molecule, respectively. However, other accessory signals are also important. Some of the other antigens important in this secondary signal include the cell adhesion molecules and B7/CD28.[52,53]

In mice and humans, the CD28-B7 interaction has been identified as a source of costimulatory signals. Consistent with this model, a soluble fusion protein of CTLA4 T-cell surface molecule with a high affinity for B7 inhibits T cell-dependent responses in vivo and in vitro. These costimulatory signals delivered by the antigen-presenting cells are critical because lack of these signals results in lack of an immune response. More specifically, these mice become tolerant to the immunogen. The B7 molecule is a costimulatory molecule that regulates IL-2 secretion through the pathway that uses CD28 and CTLA4. Recent evidence suggests that there are family of B7 molecules now termed B7-1 and B7-2 which are expressed and are distinct from each other.[54-56] B7-2 (or otherwise known as GL1) is considered the predominant counter-receptor for the T-cell activation of molecule CTLA4 and CD28. This B7-2 provides a critical signal for T cell-dependent responses in vivo and in vitro. Murine B7 is a 50-60 kd glycoprotein consisting of immunoglobulin V- and C-like extracellular domain, transmembrane region and a short cytoplasmic tail.[57] The progression from multiple costimulatory signals is unknown. Clearly, a T cell which has received the first signal from the T-cell receptor must connect within 12-24 hours either to activate an immune response or to commit itself to anergy. Further understanding of these costimulatory pathways will be important to understand autoimmunity and the control of autoimmunity, potential induction of transplantation tolerance and possibly stimulation of viral or anti-viral anti-tumor activity. Experiments with these molecules have recently shown blockage of B7 family of costimulatory molecules reducing the alloreactive precursor T cells capable of inducing GVHD.[58] There was specific inhibition of the frequency of alloreactive precursor T cells in induction of alloantigen-specific hyper-responsiveness. A second experiment used in vivo infusion of soluble CTLA4-Ig[59] reduced lethal GVHD across major histocompatibility complex barrier in mice.

These molecules help initiate T-cell responses. Several of these accessory signals may also result in the release of cytokines such as TNF, interferon-γ or IL-1.[60-61] Thus, when an immune reaction occurs, these donor-derived T cells may secrete cytokines that in turn modulate or release other cytokines down a cytokine cascade. Moreover, this cascade may result from other accessory cells than these donor-derived T cells.

## REFERENCES

1. Sayegh M, Fine NA, Smith JL, Rennke HG, Milford EL, Tilney NL. Immunologic tolerance to renal allografts after bone marrow transplants from the same donors. Ann Int Med 1991; 114: 954.
2. Beatty P, Clift RA, Mickelson EM et al. Marrow transplantation from related donors other than HLA-identical siblings. N Engl J Med 1985; 313: 765.
3. Opelz G. Correlation of HLA matching with kidney graft survival in patients with or without cyclosporine treatment. Transplantation 1985; 40: 240.
4. Hullet D, Landry AS, Leonard DK, Sollinger HW. Enhancement of thyroid allograft survival following organ culture. Alteration of tissue immunogenicity. Transplantation 1989; 47: 24.
5. Niederwieser D, Aubock J, Troppmair J et al. IFN-mediated induction of MHC antigen expression on human keratinocytes and its influence on in vitro alloimmune responses. J Immunol 1988; 140: 2556.
6. Azogui O, Gluckman E, Fradelizi D. Inhibition of IL-2 production after human allogeneic bone marrow transplantation. J Immunol 1983; 131: 1205.
7. Andrus L, Lafferty KJ. Inhibition of T-cell activity by cyclosporin A. Scand J Immunol 1982; 15: 449.
8. Reem G, Cook LA, Vilcek J. Gamma interferon synthesis by human thymocytes and T lymphocytes inhibited by cyclosporin A. Science 1983; 221: 63.
9. Storb R, Deeg HJ, Whitehead J et al. Methotrexate and cyclosporine compared with cyclosporine alone for prophylaxis of acute graft-versus-host disease after marrow transplantation for leukemia. N Engl J Med 1986; 314: 729.
10. Morecki S, Leshem B, Weigenberg M, Bar S, Slavin S. Functional clonal deletion versus active suppression in transplantation tolerance induced by total-lymphoid irradiation. Transplantation 1985; 40: 201.

11. Rosenkrantz K, Keever C, Bhimani K et al. Both on-going suppression and clonal elimination contribute to graft-host tolerance after transplantation of HLA-mismatched T-cell-depleted marrow for severe combined immunodeficiency. J Immunol 1990; 144: 1721.

12. Vallera D, Soderling CCB, Orosz CG. Assessment of immunocompetence by limiting dilution analysis in long-term T-cell depletion chimeras transplanted across the MHC barrier. Transplantation 1985; 40: 311.

13. Gebel H, Daiser H, Landay AL. Characterization of circulating suppressor T lymphocytes in bone marrow transplant recipients. Transplantation 1987; 43: 258.

14. Tsoi M, Storb R, Dobbs S, Thomas ED. Specific suppressor cells in graft-host tolerance of HLA-identical marrow transplantation. Nature 1981; 292:355.

15. Marrack P, Kappler J. The staphylococcal enterotoxins and their relatives. Science 1990; 248: 705.

16. Kappler J, Roehm N, Marrack P. T-cell tolerance by clonal elimination in the thymus. Cell 1987; 49: 272.

17. von Boehmer H, Kisielow P. Self-nonself discrimination by T cells. Science,1990; 248: 1369.

18. Sha W, Nelson CA, Newberry RD, Kranz DM, Russell JH, Loh DY. Positive and negative selection of an antigen receptor on T cells in transgenic mice. Nature 1988; 336: 73.

19. Marrack P, Lo D, Brinster R et al. The effect of thymus enviroment on T-cell development and tolerance. Cell 1988; 53: 627.

20. Schwartz R. A cell culture model for T-lymphocyte clonal anergy. Science 1990; 248: 1329.

21. Gimmi C, Freeman GJ, Gribben JG et al. B-cell surface antigen B7 provides a costimulatory signal that induces T cells to proliferate and secrete interleukin 2. Proc Natl Acad Sci 1991; 88: 6575.

22. Linsley P, Brady W, Grosmaire L, Aruffo A, Damle NK, Ledbetter JA. Binding of the B-cell activation antigen B7 to CD28 costimulates T-cell proliferation and interleukin 2 mRNA accumulation. J Exp Med 1991; 173:721.

23. Gershon RK. A disquisition on suppressor T cells. Transplant Rev 1975; 26:170.

24. Tomita Y, Mayumi H, Eto M, Nomoto K. Importance of suppressor T cells in cyclophosphamide-induced tolerance to the non-H-2-encoded alloantigens. Is mixed chimerism really required in maintaining a skin allograft tolerance. J Immunol 1990; 144: 463.

25. Roser B. Cellular mechanisms in neonatal and adult tolerance. Immunol Rev 1989; 107: 179.

26. Tutschka P, Ki PF, Beschorner WE, Hess AD, Santos GW. Suppressor cells in transplantation tolerance. II. Maturation of suppressor cells in the bone marrow chimera. Transplantation 1981; 32: 321.

27. Wilson D. Idiotypic regulation of T cells in graft-versus-host disease and autoimmunity. Immunol Rev 1989; 107: 159.

28. Palathumpa V, Dejbakhsh-Jones S, Holm B, Strober S. Different subsets of T cells in the adult mouse bone marrow and spleen induce or suppress acute graft-versus-host disease. J Immunol 1992; 149: 808.

29. Sugiura K, Inaba M, Ogata H et al. Wheat germ agglutinin-positive cells in a stem cell-enriched fraction of mouse bone marrow have potent natural suppressor activity. Proc Natl Acad Sci 1988; 85: 4824.

30. Sugiura K, Ikehara S, Gengozian N et al. Enrichment of natural suppressor activity in a wheat germ agglutinin positive hematopoietic progenitor-enriched fraction of monkey bone marrow. Blood 1990; 75: 1125.

31. Maier T, Holda JH, Claman HN. Natural suppressor (NS) cells. Members of the LGL regulatory family. Immunol Today 1986; 7: 312.

32. Holda J, Maier T, Claman HN. Evidence that IFN-γ is responsible for natural suppressor activity in GVHD spleen and normal bone marrow. Transplantation 1988 45: 772.

33. Pourshadi M, De Fazio SR, Gozzo JJ. Suppression of second set rejection of skin allografts by donor bone marrow cells. Transpl Proc 1989; 21: 264.

34. Miller R, Muraoka S, Claesson MH, Reimann J, Benveniste P. The veto phenomenon in T-cell regulation. Ann NY Acad Sci 1988; 532: 170.

35. Heeg K, Wagner H. Induction of peripheral tolerance to class I major histocompatibility complex (MHC) alloantigens in adult mice: Transfused class I MHC-incompatible splenocytes veto clonal response of antigen-reactive Lyt-2+ T cells. J Exp Med 1988; 172: 719.

36. Azuma E, Yamamoto H, Kaplan J. Use of lymphokine-activated keller cells to prevent bone marrow graft rejection and lethal graft-versus-host disease. J Immunol 1989; 143: 1524.

37. Knulst A, Bril-Bazuin C, Tibbe GJM, Benner R. Improved survival from potentially lethal graft-vs.-host disease by donor pretreatment with a recipient-specific blood transfusion: I. Requirements for induction and specificity of the effect. Eur J Immunol 1992; 22: 2481.

38. Hiruma K, Gress RE. Cyclosporine A and peripheral tolerance. Inhibition of veto cell-mediated clonal deletion of postthymic precursor cytotoxic T lymphocytes. J Immunol 1992; 149: 1539.

39. Sykes M, Chester CH, Sachs D. Protection from graft-versus-host disease in fully allogeneic chimeras by prior administration of T-cell-depleted syngeneic bone marrow. Transplantation 1988; 46: 327.

40. Sykes M, Eisenthal A, Sachs DH. Mechanism of protection from graft-versus-host disease in murine mixed allogeneic chimeras. J Immunol 1988.140: 2903.

41. Sykes M, Sharabi Y, Sachs DH. Achieving alloengraftment without graft-versus-host disease: Approaches using mixed allogeneic bone marrow transplantation. Bone Marrow Transpl 1988; 3: 379.

42. Sykes M, Chester CH, Sundt TM, Romick ML, Hoyles KA, Sachs DH. Effects of T-cell depletion in radiation bone marrow chimeras. J Immunol 1989; 143: 3503.

43. Ramsdell F, Lantz T, Fowlkes BJ. A nondeletional mechanism of thymic self tolerance. Science 1989; 246: 1038.

44. Yazdi B, Patel MP, Ramsamooj R et al. Vascularized bone marrow transplantation (VBMT): Induction of stable mixed T-cell chimerism and tranplantation tolerance in unmodified recipients. Transpl Proc 1991 23: 739.

45. Waer M, Vandeputte M. Allogeneic thymus transplantation as a means to induce transplantation tolerance. Transpl Proc 1990; 22: 1970.

46. Billingham R, Brent L, Medawar PB. Actively acquired tolerance of grafted cells. Nature 1953; 239: 603.

47. Gowans J, McGregor DD, Cowen DM, Ford CE. Initiation of responses by small lymphocytes. Nature 1962 196: 651.

48. Silvers W. Studies on the apparent serial passage of transplantation immunity in tolerant mice. Transplantation 1980; 10: 538.

49. Wren S, Hronakes ML, Ildstad ST. CD4⁺ T cells, but not CD8⁺ T cells, mediate the breaking of tolerance in mixed allogeneic chimeras (B10⁺ B10.BR → B10). Transplantation 1993; 55: 1382.

50. Perreault C, Belanger R, Gyger M. Allard A, Brochu S. The mechanism of graft-host-tolerance in murine radiation chimeras transplanted across minor histocompatibility barriers. Bone Marrow Transpl 1989; 4: 83.

51. Perreault C, Allard A, Brochu S et al. Studies of immunologic tolerance to host minor histocompatibility antigens following allogeneic bone marrow transplantation in mice. Bone Marrow Transpl 1990; 6: 127.

52. Koulova L, Clark EA, Shu G, Dupont B. The CD28 ligand B7/BB1 provides costimulatory signal for alloactivation of CD4⁺ T cells. J Exp Med 1991; 173: 759.

53. Simon J, Cruz PD, Tigelaar RE, Sontheimer RD, Bergstresser PR. Adhesion molecules CD11a, CD18; and ICAM-1 on human epidermal Langerhans cells serve a functional role in the activation of alloreactive T cells. J Invest Dermatol 1991; 96: 148.

54. Hathcock K, Laszlo G, Dicker HB, Bradshaw J, Linsley P, Hodes RJ. Identification of an alternative CTLA-4 ligand costimulatory for T-cell activation. Science 1993; 262: 905.

55. Freeman G, Borriello F, Hodes RJ et al. Uncovering of functional alternative CTLA-4 counter-receptor in B7-deficient mice. Science 1993; 262: 907.

56. Freeman G, Gribben JG, Boussiotis VA et al. Cloning of B7-2: A CTLA-4 counter-receptor that costimulates human T-cell proliferation. Science 1993; 209: 909.

57. Freeman G, Gray GS, Gimmi CD et al. Structure, expression, and T cell costimulatory activity of the murine homologue of the human B lymphocyte activation antigen B7. J Exp Med 1991; 174: 625.

58. Gribben J, Boussiotis V, Freeman G, Gray G, Nadler L. Blockade of the B7 family of costimulatory molecules significantly reduces alloreactive precursor T cells capable of inducing GVHD. Blood 1993; 82 (Suppl 1): 456a.

59. Blazar B, Taylor PA, Linsley PS, Varella DA. In vivo infusion of soluble CTLA4-Ig reduces lethal graft-versus-host disease (GVHD) induced across the major histocompatibility complex (MHC) barrier in mice. Blood 1993; 82 (suppl 1): 456a.

60. Unanue E, Allen PM. The basis for the immunoregulatory role of macrophages and other accessory cells. Science 1987; 236: 551.

61. Scheurich P, Thoma B, Ucer U, Pfizenmaier K. Immunoregulatory activity of recombinant tumor necrosis factor induction of TNF receptors on human T cells and TNF-α mediated enhancement of T-cell responses. J Immunol 1987; 138: 1786.

# CHAPTER 7

# CLINICAL ASPECTS OF ACUTE GRAFT-VERSUS-HOST DISEASE

## CLINICAL AND HISTOLOGIC MANIFESTATIONS

### SKIN

As described earlier, many manifestations of GVHD in humans are analogous to those observed in animals. Usually, the first (and most common) clinical manifestation of acute GVHD is a maculopapular skin rash, usually occurring at or near the time of the white blood cell engraftment (Fig. 7.1). The early stages of this rash may be pruritic, involving the nape of the neck, ears and shoulders as well as the palms of the hands and the soles of the feet. This rash can also be described as a sunburn. From these initial areas of presentation, the rash may spread to involve the whole integument and becomes confluent. In severe GVHD, the maculopapular rash forms bulbous lesions with epidermal necrolysis. The progression of GVHD can be clinically defined into four stages depending on the extent of involvement of the skin (Table 7.1).

The histologic changes of GVHD of the skin involve dermal and epidermal changes.[1,2] Several characteristic findings include exocytosed lymphocytes, dyskeratotic epidermal keratinocytes, follicular involvement, satellite lymphocytes adjacent to or surrounding dyskeratotic epidermal keratinocytes and dermal perivascular lymphocytic infiltration.[3] The most consistent histologic feature is individual cell necrosis (apoptosis) at the base of crypts (Fig. 7.2). However, similar changes can be seen from cytotoxic therapy as used in the preparative regimen for BMT and with infections. One possible marker for GVHD is an increase in HLA-DR expression in keratinocytes.[4] Staining for the DR antigen has produced variable results.[5] A recent study evaluated the distribution of two cellular adhesion molecules, ELAM-1 and VCAM-1.[6] VCAM-1 positivity was seen on a few endothelial cells in normal skin, but was mainly observed on dermal dendritic cells surrounding blood vessels and adnexal structures. In specimens with GVHD, there was an increase in positive dendritic cells and the appearance of a large number of similar cells throughout the upper epidermis. Fortunately, skin GVHD, if not progressing to other organ disease, responds to treatment for acute GVHD.

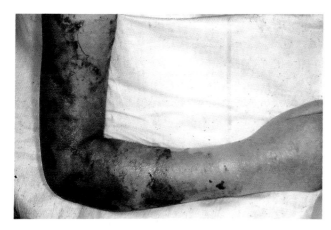

Fig. 7.1. Clinical appearance of a patient with severe skin GVHD. Note the generalized erythroderma and formation of bullae.

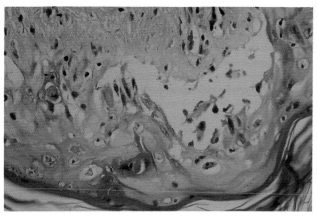

Fig. 7.2. Histologic appearance of the skin reflecting the clinical changes with disruption of the dermal-epidermal junction.

### Table 7.1. GVHD grading of individual organ systems

| Organ | Grade | Description |
|-------|-------|-------------|
| Skin | +1 | Maculopapular eruption over <25% of body area |
|  | +2 | Maculopapular eruption over 35-50% of body area |
|  | +3 | Generalized erythroderma |
|  | +4 | Generalized erythroderma with bullous formation and often with desquamation |
| Liver | +1 | Bilirubin 2.0-3.0 mg/dl; SGOT 150-750 IU |
|  | +2 | Bilirubin 3.1-6.0 mg/dl |
|  | +3 | Bilirubin 6.1-15.0 mg/dl |
|  | +4 | Bilirubin > 15.0 mg/dl |
| Gut | +1 | Diarrhea > 30 ml/kg or 500 ml/day |
|  | +2 | Diarrhea > 60 ml/kg or 1000 ml/day |
|  | +3 | Diarrhea > 90 ml/kg or 1500 ml/day |
|  | +4 | Diarrhea > 90 ml/kg or 2000 ml/day or severe abdominal pain or ileus |

Adapted from Glucksberg et al (ref. 12).

Studies of cutaneous acute GVHD have shown that the dermal lymphocytes are composed almost entirely of T cells with a relative predominance of CD4[+] cells, whereas epidermal lymphocytes exhibit a comparatively striking predominance of the suppressor subset CD8[+] cells.[7] Using an antibody termed HECA-452, which has been found to identify a subet of T lymphocytes that display preferential localization to the skin, investigators have been able to study histologically the presence of T cells in acute GVHD. Results demonstrate that T lymphocytes expressing HECA-452 epitope are present in cutaneous GVHD but not in GVHD found in other organs. Further characterization of skin infiltrating T lymphocytes during acute GVHD has been carried out studying a panel of 34 clones established from a cell line derived from the skin biopsy of a patient undergoing acute GVHD after semi-allogeneic bone marrow transplantation (bone marrow donated by the father).[8] All but one of the 34 clones obtained were the CD4[+] phenotype and none were CD16[+]. Only the sole CD8[+] clone showed significant cytotoxicity against the father's hemoglutin and blast.

Immunohistochemical analyses of skin biopsies from allogeneic BMT recipients with either acute GVHD or chronic GVHD were studied using a panel of different monoclonal antibodies.[9] Included in the panel of antibodies was a novel NK-associated cell surface antigen (Kp43). This data indicated that, in the GVHD lesions, the proportion of CD2[+] cells often exceeded those detected with anti-CD3 monoclonal antibodies. Double labeling confirmed the presence of CD2[+] CD3[-] lymphocytes. Again, no CD16[+] lymphocytes were observed. However, most samples consistently displayed a substantial portion of the Kp43[+] cells. Use of this novel antigen may allow discussion of questions involving the importance of NK cells in the effector phase of GVHD. This study suggests that these NK cells may be secondarily attracted to the skin by antigen-specific T cells.[10]

## LIVER

The liver is the second most commonly involved organ by acute GVHD. Rarely, patients will have moderate to severe liver GVHD without evidence of cutaneous disease. Liver involvement is manifest by abnormal liver function tests and is difficult to treat effectively. The earliest and most common abnormality is a rise in the conjugated bilirubin and alkaline phosphatase. This reflects the pathology associated with liver GVHD, that is, damage to the bile canaliculi leading to cholestasis. Unfortunately, a rise in the bilirubin or alkaline phosphatase is far from specific. There are many competing factors that may lead to abnormal liver function tests. Common competing factors include: veno-occlusive disease of the liver (a relatively common toxicity associated with the use of high dose therapy), hepatic infections (primarily viral), effects from the preparatory regimen and drug toxicity including the drugs used for GVHD prophylaxis (cyclosporine and/or methotrexate). The most definitive method to diagnose GVHD of the liver is by biopsy. This may not be feasible, primarily due to concerns of acute bleeding which can be significant early after BMT. Newer approaches, such as a transjugular approach, may be better suited methods for the biopsy if an adequate amount of tissue is obtained. The primary histologic finding (Fig. 7.3) is that of bile duct atypia and degeneration leading occasionally to severe cholestasis.[11]

## GASTROINTESTINAL TRACT

The third main organ system to be affected by GVHD is the gut. Gut GVHD is often the most severe and also difficult to treat. Gut GVHD is characterized by diarrhea and abdominal cramping. The diarrhea can be quite voluminous so that it becomes difficult to maintain an adequate fluid balance in some patients. The crampy abdominal pain associated with severe GVHD can also be quite difficult to treat. A severe ileus may develop associated with the GVHD or with increased narcotic use to control the physical discomfort. The amount of diarrhea in some patients can be in excess of 10 liters per day (Table 7.1). The diarrhea may be watery initially, reflecting primarily salt and water re-absorption defect in the distal small bowel and colon, but frequently becomes bloody so that transfusion requirements can be quite significant.[12] It is not unusual for patients to need two units of packed red blood cells nearly daily to keep up the hematocrit in the 30% range. The stages of gut GVHD are usually graded by the volume of diarrhea. There is one caveat, however, and that is that diarrhea is a very common occurrence following BMT. Within the first weeks, the diarrhea may be related to the preparatory regimen, the nonabsorbable antibiotics or the systemic antibiotics. Later in the course of BMT, superinfection must be considered as a cause for the diarrhea as well as Clostitium difficile toxin. Histologically in GVHD, the gut shows crypt cell necrosis.[11] Degenerative material accumulates in these dead crypts (Fig. 7.4). There is

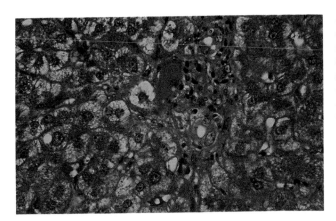

*Fig. 7.3. Histologic appearance of the liver showing bile duct atypia and degeneration. These changes can occasionally lead to severe cholestasis.*

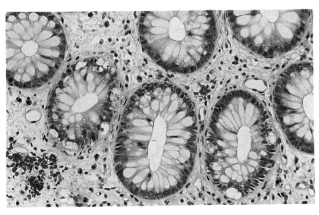

*Fig. 7.4. Histologic apperance of gut pathology demonstrating crypt necrosis and dead cells.*

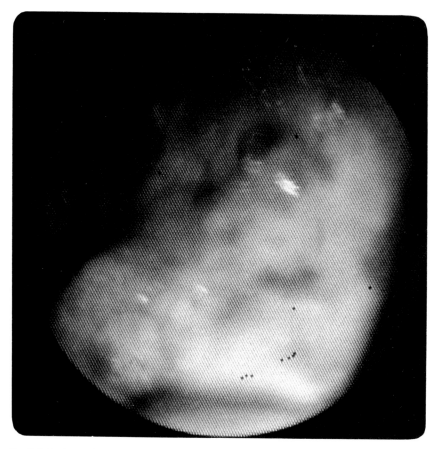

*Fig. 7.5. Endoscopic appearance of the duodenum in a patient with acute GVHD.*

extensive destruction of these crypts leading to crypt drop-out and loss of crypt throughout the affected areas. In cases of severe gut GVHD, there may be whole areas that are denuded with total loss of the epithelium similar to that observed in the skin. A rectal biopsy is usually helpful in making the diagnosis of gut GVHD. Colonoscopy or upper endoscopy is usually also performed (Fig. 7.5). However, infectious agents, most notoriously cytomegalovirus may mimic clinical as well as histological features of acute GVHD in the gut. Selective staining for such pathogens should be pursued to rule out the possibility that an infectious agent is the cause of the gastrointestinal symptoms. A recent study evaluated the distribution of three cellular adhesion molecules, ICAM-1, ELAM-1 and VCAM-1.[13] Although VCAM-1 expression was significantly increased in the skin, a similar increase was not found in enterocytes. This study concluded it was unlikely that immunostaining for these adhesion molecules would be useful for the diagnosis of GVHD. An interesting observation has been made that nitric oxide mediates the intestinal pathology in GVHD.[14] Using a specific inhibitor of nitric oxide, L-N$^G$-monomethyl arginine (L-NMMA), these authors abolished, in a dose-dependent manner, the crypt hypertrophy and hyperplasia that usually occurs in the intestine of mice with GVHD. There was significant decrease in the lymphocytic infiltration of the epithelium. However, nitric oxide does not appear to affect the induction of GVHD since the accompanying splenomegaly was not affected. The actual mechanism of action of nitric oxide remains to be elucidated.

A group at the University of Minnesota has also described an entity of acute upper GI GVHD.[15] This form of acute GVHD presents clinically with anorexia, dyspepsia, food intolerance, nausea and vomiting. This syndrome was recognized and documented by upper endoscopic biopsies of the esophagus and stomach, and seems to be more responsive to immunosuppressive treatment. Patients failing the treatment for upper GI GVHD progress to symptomatic lower GI GVHD, suggesting that this syndrome may be an earlier, and perhaps more treatable, form of intestinal pathology. Interestingly, those with this syndrome of upper GI acute GVHD were significantly older than the overall BMT population and older than the cohort with overall grade II-IV GVHD.

## HEMATOLYMPHOID ORGAN

Although the hematolymphoid organ is not commonly considered in acute GVHD, the ravages of GVHD are expressed in this organ system. Early studies of GVHD, recognized that the brunt of the graft-versus-host reaction occurred in the host lymphoid organs.[12] As a consequence, the hosts' immune competence was affected, leading to frequent and possibly fatal infectious complications. A profound drop in immunoglobulins was often observed. GVHD may also affect hematopoiesis, leading to a reduction of hematopoietic cells.[16] Although there was not a clear decrease in the peripheral blood counts in murine models, the number of hematopoietic precursors remained low. In humans, following BMT, the effect of GVHD on the hematopoietic system is usually not dramatic. However, persistent thrombocytopenia is a frequent manifestation of GVHD. The presence of active GVHD may not only be immunosuppressive but may also decrease responsiveness to active immunization. One study suggests that immune responses to polio vaccination resulted in less protection in those patients who had graft-versus-host disease.[17]

## OVERALL GRADE

Each stage of each organ involvement is combined to obtain an overall grade of acute GVHD (Table 7.2). Clinically significant acute GVHD is

### Table 7.2. Overall grading of acute GVHD

| Grade | Skin | Liver | | Gut | ECOG Performance |
|-------|------|-------|---|-----|------------------|
| I | +1 to +2 | 0* | | 0 | 0 |
| II | +1 to +3 | +1 | and/or | +1 | 0-1 |
| III | +2 to +3 | +2 to +4 | and/or | +2 to +3 | 2-3 |
| IV | +2 to +4 | +2 to +4 | and/or | +2 to +4 | 3-4 |

*The original Glucksberg grading allowed for +1 liver involvement in overall grade I GVHD.

usually defined as overall grade II to grade IV acute GVHD. Grade I GVHD is defined as mild GVHD, grade II GVHD as moderate and grade III-IV as severe GVHD.[12] Overall grading is important in terms of assessing response to prophylaxis or treatment, impact on survival and association with graft-versus-leukemia effect. Patients with moderate to severe GVHD have a significantly higher mortality rate. One difficulty with organ stage involvement and the overall grading of acute GVHD is that most of the initial reports and observations described were before the cyclosporine era.[18] Initial GVHD prophylaxis involved the use of single agents such as methotrexate or cyclophosphamide. The emerging picture of acute GVHD in the cyclosporine era, and with combinations of the single agents, may present a different sequence of events even though the overall organ manifestations are the same. That is, there are now patients with single organ stage IV GVHD who would not fit into the overall schema for grade IV GVHD, although nearly all investigators would agree that such a patient has severe GVHD. On the other hand, a patient with just skin GVHD, even if grade IV skin GVHD, would be expected to have a much more favorable outcome than a patient with grade IV gut GVHD, even though the two would both have overall grade IV GVHD. Because of this discrepancy, several investigators have attempted to create a staging of acute GVHD that gives both prognostic information and allows for comparisons.[19] Unfortunately, a new staging system has not found widespread usage.

An example of the difficulty in diagnosis and grading of acute GVHD was reflected in a study conducted by the International Bone Marrow Transplant Registry.[20] Six clinical vignettes were evaluated by 49 transplant physicians from 42 bone marrow transplant centers worldwide. The concordance for the diagnosis of acute GVHD ranged from 24-74% and the concordance for grading the GVHD was 55%. The concordance for the decision to treat for acute GVHD ranged from 43-55% and the concordance for assigning the primary cause of death was 71-100%. These results underscore the need for revision of the scoring criteria as diagnostic methods and knowledge of the disease improves.

## OTHER MANIFESTATIONS

Murine models of GVHD suggest that the production of potentially pathogenic IgG antinuclear antibodies is not sufficient for the development of renal disease in lupus-like nephritis. This suggests that a separate event from autoantibody production is MHC-dependent and appears to be critical for the formation and/or deposition of pathologic immune complexes. Murine data show the development of severe nephritis and autoantibody production depends on the MHC type of the recipient.[21] That is, some mice will develop severe nephrotic syndrome leading to death, in contrast to other mice where a high level of autoantibodies are produced but progression to renal failure was not observed. These studies show the importance of class II molecules in determining the outcome of such a graft-versus-host reaction. A striking difference among the graft-versus-host combinations appeared to be at the level of deposition or formation of immune complexes within the glomeruli.

Patients undergoing BMT can be considered infants based on the distribution pattern of specific serum antibodies that appears after BMT.[22]

Moreover, IgG (especially IgG2 and IgG4) and low IgA levels are found in a large proportion of long-term survivors after BMT. In childhood, there is an increase in IgG1 and IgG3, but levels of IgG2, IgG4 and IgA levels may not reach normal levels until puberty. Various investigators demonstrated that IgA deficiency occurs in many patients following allogeneic BMT.[23,24] This deficiency seems to be related to the development of acute and chronic GVHD.[25] A review of 131 patients undergoing allogeneic BMT found that acute GVHD was a predisposing factor for the development of IgA deficiency.[26] Prophylaxis for acute GVHD also influenced the development of IgA deficiency, but the development of acute GVHD was not essential for IgA deficiency.

An increase in IgE levels following allogeneic bone marrow transplantation has been described by several investigators.[27] This has been found in the majority of patients with acute GVHD and lead to the suggestion that increased IgE synthesis may be related to an imbalance in T-cell regulation that occurs during GVHD. However, these levels seem to be highest in syngeneic recipients, thereby suggesting that there is not a direct relationship between post-BMT IgE synthesis and GVHD.

## RISK FACTORS

There have been many retrospective analyses of the risk factors for the occurrence of GVHD. Moreover, with more effective prophylaxis regimens, especially since the introduction of cyclosporine and combinations of drug prophylaxis, the importance of each risk factor can change. These risk factors are summarized in Table 7.3.

### HLA Discrepancy

From early animal studies to more recent matched unrelated donor transplantation, one paramount factor is the degree of HLA disparity. The initial data presented will relate only to genotypically related donor transplantation. However, in recipients of matched unrelated donor transplantation, HLA typing, specifically molecular matching, is critical in decreasing the incidence of GVHD. The Seattle BMT group reviewed their experience with HLA-mismatched recipients.[28] The incidence of GVHD for those patients with genotypic 1-3 antigen mismatch was approximately double compared to the matched recipients. Phenotypically matched family

---

*Table 7.3. Risk factors for acute GVHD*

HLA disparity
Age
Donor: recipient gender
Donor: recipient parity
Type of disease
Disease status
Dose of radiation
Dose of methotrexate and cyclosporine delivered
? sterile enviroment (including gut decontamination)
? HLA haplotype

member recipients had the same incidence when compared to genotypically matched recipients.

There are some suggestions, albeit preliminary, that DP matching may be correlated with a higher incidence of severe acute GVHD in recipients of BMT from unrelated donors.[29] This data remains controversial, as other studies have not noted the importance of DP in matched unrelated donor transplantation. Some of these dichotomies may be related to initial lack of PCR typing of the D or DR regions. Fine DNA typing may explain some of these inconsistencies. However, observations of extended haplotypes do suggest that DP is not highly correlated with HLA, A, B and DR.

## AGE

Age is a second important factor commonly associated with an increase risk of GVHD.[30-32] The clearest example is a comparison of the incidence of GVHD between pediatric and adult patients. It is unclear if this difference is due to the age of the recipient or possibly the age of the donor. Since BMT is common for matched sibling donors most of the donor-recipient pairs are close in age. There may be a propensity to a higher incidence of GVHD because of immunological factors associated with aging, such as increase antigen sensitization or thymic involution.

## GNOTOBIOSIS

A third important factor from animal studies is the influence of environmental factors related primarily to infections. Gnotobiotic (germ-free) environment is a highly successful approach in experimental murine systems.[33,34] The mechanism for this protection is unknown, but may be secondary to cross-reactive antigens between bacterial or viral pathogens or to cytokine released in response to infections which may recruit alloresponsive cells. Compared to conventionally treated mice, the incidence and mortality from GVHD was considerably lower in the germ-free mice. If these mice are colonized with a single strain of gram-negative bacteria, GVHD ensues. In clinical trials gnotobiosis is associated with improved outcome in patients undergoing BMT for aplastic anemia.[35] It is less likely to help those patients undergoing BMT for leukemias. It appears to be difficult, if not clinically impossible, to approach the gnotobiotic environment found in murine models. The primary difficulty is the sterilization of the gut and skin flora despite use of potent antibiotics.

Suppression of intestinal flora, specifically the anaerobic bacteria, seems to reduce the risk of acute GVHD. One study analyzed 194 patients following genotypically identical BMT.[36] These patients were under strict protective isolation and intestinal antimicrobial decontamination. Of 45 patients (23%) who developed acute GVHD, a multivariate analysis revealed that one of the factors associated with the occurrence of GVHD was ineffective suppression of intestinal anaerobic bacteria evidenced by sustained growth of these anaerobic bacteria in cultures. The duration of anaerobic growth suppression as a time-dependent variable in a proportional hazard regression analysis confirmed this feature as an independent predictor for acute GVHD. This study, however, used extensive oral decontamination with 320 mg of gentamicin or tobramycin or 600 mg of netilmycin in combination with 2,800 mg of amphotericin B and $5.2 \times 10^6$ U nystatin administered orally divided into four doses daily. Some patients also received four daily oral doses of 500 mg of cefazolin solution. If analyses of fecal samples indicated colonization of the gastrointestinal tract with bacteria resistant to the decontamination medications, additional treatment with oral or parenteral antibiotics was initiated according to the results of sensitivity testing. All patients were housed in filtered air rooms, as well as strict isolation and oral decontamination and skin cleansing using 1-propanol, 2-propanol and 2-biphenylol disinfection of the skin and disinfection of the oral mucous membranes using polyvinyl-pyrrolidon-iodine solution three times daily. The hypothesis tested was that increased lymphokine secretion stimulated by endotoxin or other bacterial products might lead to nonspecific activation and polyclonal expansion of graft-derived T cells. These T cells could then promote a specific allogeneic response to donor lymphocytes against nonshared histocompatibility antigen recipient tissue. Experimental evidence from murine studies suggests that allorecognition of donor T lymphocytes may be induced by cross-reactions between intestinal bacterial antigens and the antigens of the mucosa epithelium.[37] Another study in the pediatric patient population showed similar results, suggesting that complete gastrointestinal decontamination in a strict protective environment was an effective method of preventing severe infections in acute GVHD.[38]

## HLA-Linkage

The linkage with certain HLA types is intriguing and was reported previously.[32,39] The first study reported an increased risk of GVHD associated with HLA-B18 along with a reduced risk associated with HLA-B8, BW35 and B15. There was, however, a 2.06-fold increase in GVHD associated with A26, along with A10 and A25. Unfortunately, the class II antigens were not examined in this study. The second study found a higher incidence of GVHD associated with AW19 and cross-reactive antigens 29, 30, 31 or 33, CW4 and BW21, 49 or 50. A third study reported recently suggested an association between HLA-B alleles and protection from GVHD.[40] The relevant gene lies between HLA-A and HLA-DR but is not DR2, and is close to HLA-B. Genes mapped to this region include TNF and HSP70. Experimental murine data show strains of mice are high or low producers of TNF and that this characteristic is associated with susceptibility to autoimmune states such as lupus nephritis. Both of these genes may play a central role in the pathogenesis of acute GVHD. A recent study also found an association between HLA-DR4 and chronic GVHD in the South Wales population.[41] It remains unclear if these associations are still based on chance or on unique immunologic phenomena as is seen with certain autoimmune diseases.

## Gender/Parity

Two recent reviews have stratified the risk factors associated with the occurrence of GVHD.[30,31] The first study from the Minnesota BMT group analyzed patients from both the pre- and post-cyclosporine era. In the univariate analysis, age, donor:recipient sex match, female:female transplants, and HLA-DR3 were associated with less GVHD. More frequent GVHD was associated with BMT for chronic myelogenous leukemia, cytomegalovirus seropositivity, prior donor allosensitization (pregnancy or transfusions), and the presence of the HLA-A26 allele.[30] A stepwise multivariate analysis confirmed the importance of increased age, donor:recipient gender (not female:female) and the protective effect of HLA-DR3.

The second study investigated patients from a single institution who received marrow grafts from HLA identical siblings and prophylaxis for GVHD consisting of cyclosporine and methotrexate—a relatively uniform group of patients.[31] The incidence of grade II-IV acute GVHD was 35%. In the univariate analysis the factors associated with increased risk for acute GVHD were: increasing patient age, increasing donor age, patient:donor sex mismatch and female parity. In a multivariate analysis, recipient-donor sex and parity were the most significant predictive factors; donor or recipient age did not add to the predictive value. Disease status prior to BMT and the dose of total body irradiation were also important in assessing the risk for GVHD. Patients with more advanced disease had a higher risk of GVHD as did those who received more than 1,200 cGy of total body irradiation. Delivery of full doses of methotrexate and cyclosporine were also associated with a lower relative risk of developing acute GVHD. Moreover, full doses of cyclosporine resulted in less severe GVHD among patients who developed GVHD. The maintenance of full doses of cyclosporine was more predictive than serum cyclosporine levels. This is in contrast to an earlier report from the same group that described an association between cyclosporine levels and the occurrence of GVHD.[42] This earlier study had indicated that low cyclosporine concentrations could be a cause of treatment failure. The report by Nash et al also did not find any correlation between either the donor or the recipient cytomegalovirus or herpes simplex serology. Patients treated in laminar air flow rooms had the same incidence of acute GVHD as did patients not in laminar air flow rooms. No clear association was found for patient HLA antigens although the data presented only focused on selected HLA-A and B antigens. One other factor was predictive for acute GVHD in this study: year of transplantation ($\leq$1987 versus 1988). There was no good explanation for this finding.

## OTHER

The role of splenectomy in the incidence of very acute GVHD was investigated 157 patients with diverse diagnoses who had undergone HLA-matched transplantation with T-cell depletion in France.[43] Thirty-one patients (20%) had been splenectomized before transplantation. In the univariate analyses, three significant risk factors were linked with the occurrence of GVHD: splenectomy, age of recipient and GVHD prevention by monotherapy versus a combination of methotrexate and cyclosporine. Multivariate analysis demonstrated that splenectomy was a most important factor in GVHD severity. One explanation for the adverse effect of splenectomy could be the spleen's possible function as a filter of active T lymphocytes from the transplant.

The effects of pretransplant herpes virus serology in the occurrence of grade II-IV GVHD was studied in 262 recipients and the HLA identical donor.[44] In 131 recipients receiving either methotrexate or cyclosporine, significant effects were observed for the donor HSV serology with seropositivity being associated with increased risk of GVHD. Moreover, donor seronegativity for EBV was associated with increased risk of GVHD. However, these effects were nonsignificant in the other 131 recipients who received a more intensive GVHD prophylactic regimen such as methotrexate, cyclosporine A and in vivo anti-T-cell monoclonal antibodies or various procedures to reduce the T-cell numbers in transplants.

## PREDICTIVE TESTS

### MIXED LYMPHOCYTE CULTURE

There have been several attempts to develop assays that would predict the occurrence of acute GVHD prior to allogeneic BMT. Probably the most frequently utilized test is the mixed lymphocyte culture (MLC). The MLC is an in vitro test that measures a primary immune response of T-cell recognition and proliferation. MLR reactivity correlates with GVH reactivity, but this proliferative assay does not always predict development of GVHD in vivo, especially in MHC compatible combinations.[45] Significant MLC reactivity is usually not observed when the cells tested are from genotypically identical siblings. Reactivity, when it occurs, seems to be associated with leukemia-associated antigens.[46-50] However, a re-analysis of this method by using a significantly lower cut-off for reactivity (usually 15%), may allow for a higher predictive value of this test.[51] One difficulty with studies using the MLC has been the lack of a standardized cut-off for reactivity. Another explanation for MLC reactivity may be ascribed to unrecognized intra-HLA-D region recombination in either the donor or the recipient or in other histocompatibility antigens that have yet to be defined.

A large analysis of the MLC reactivity was undertaken in Seattle, where 783 bone marrow recipients from HLA genotypically identical sibling donors were analyzed. A greater than expected response was elicited in 10.6% of patients, with greater responses in relapsed patients compared to those in remission. Recent transfusions did not appear to affect the MLC results. No association was found between increased donor anti-recipient MLC reactivity and the subsequent development of acute GVHD. These data suggest that the MLC responses do not represent genetic differences between the donor and the host that are able to cause GVHD. Since all these patients were genotypically matched, the occurrence of GVHD would be secondary to minor histocompatibility antigen mismatches. These weaker antigenic differences are not detectable when assayed in a primary immune response test such as the MLC. However, human lymphocytes reactive to minor histocompatibility antigens can be identified in some patients such as those following cloning by limiting dilution.[52]

Following a similar line of investigation, Johnsen et al reasoned that quantitation of in vitro studies of T cell-mediated immune responses could predict for GVHD.[53,54] In vitro studies of T-cell responses have demonstrated that viral, bacterial or other antigens may mimic self HLA antigens so that they are recognized by alloreactive T cells. Donor lymphocytes were studied in 27 patients, in terms of their response to monocyte-dependent soluble antigens and to alloantigens expressed on a B-lymphoblastoid cell line. The donors were divided into high and low responders. High or low responders to soluble antigens did not correlate with the occurrence of acute GVHD. However, the responder status of the donor cells did correlate with the occurrence of GVHD. Of the 9 low responders, 3 developed acute GVHD (grade I-II) compared to the 18 high responders where 13 patients developed acute GVHD (9: grade II-IV; 4: grade I). Because of the small numbers of patients involved, this study did not achieve statistical significance.

## PRIMED MIXED LYMPHOCYTE CULTURE

A more useful tool to predict for GVHD comes from a secondary immune response in the form a skin explant model, which has been shown to have an 85% predictive rate of GVHD.[55,56] In this model, donor lymphocytes are first sensitized by using irradiated recipient lymphocytes. These donor lymphocytes are then cocultured with recipient skin in an explant. If changes are seen in the explant similar to clinical GVHD, it is considered a positive result. In those positive tests, only total removal of CD3 cells prevents the histopathology. Moreover, the CD4+ population caused the greatest degree of GVHD in vitro and direct skin infiltration by cells is not required for the skin abnormalities to become evident. This suggests that soluble factors such as cytokines are important in the effector arm of GVHD. A similar assay is the mixed epidermal cell-lymphocyte reaction.[57] Here, epidermal cells are obtained from the recipient and disaggregated by trypsin. These cells are then cocultured with donor and recipient lymphocytes similar to a MLC assay. The mixed epidermal cell-lymphocyte reaction was found to be the most predictive factor of acute GVHD as well as the severity of GVHD in a small trial.[58] These results suggest that pretransplant in vitro immune status may be used to predict for GVHD.

## SOLUBLE MHC MOLECULES

Membrane bound MHC class I molecules are restriction elements for CD8+ cytotoxic T cells. MHC class I and CD8 antigens interact in a receptor-ligand-like fashion.[59] Soluble class I antigens are found in almost all body fluids. A study has assessed the increase in soluble HLA-A, B, C with patients with ongoing GVHD.[60] This study suggests that the increase in soluble HLA, A, B and C precedes the first clinical signs of acute GVHD. These soluble markers may, therefore, be a useful indicator for the occurrence of GVHD. Other factors such as viral infections or immunosuppressive therapy may also affect the level of soluble HLA. A similar study has evaluated the serum class II levels in BMT patients compared to normal patients.[61] These levels appeared to be higher in pretransplant patients compared to healthy individuals, and in most patients, the levels rose even higher at four weeks posttransplantation. The results suggest that measurement of class II serum levels may be used for monitoring GVHD in BMT patients. However, there was a large overlap between the range of class II levels, decreasing the prognostic value. It would be necessary to collect serial blood specimens for a more complete picture. Further studies on whether these molecules could be used for predictive purposes or for monitoring response to therapy will be interesting.

# REFERENCES

1. Sale G, Lerner KG, Barker A, Shulman HM, Thomas ED. The skin biopsy in the diagnosis of acute graft-versus-host disease in man. Am J Pathol 1977; 89: 621.

2. Lerner K, Kao GF, Storb R, Buckner CD, Clift RA, Thomas ED. Histopathology of graft-versus-host reaction (GVHR) in human recipients of marrow from HLA-matched sibling donors. Transplant Proc 1974; 6: 1974.

3. Darmstat G, Donnenberg AD, Vogelsang GB, Farmer ER, Horn TD. Clinical, laboratory and histopathologic indicators of the development of progressive acute graft-versus-host disease. J Invest Dermatol 1992; 99: 397.

4. Sviland L, Pearson ADJ, Green MA et al. Class II antigen expression by keratinocytes and enterocytes is an early feature of graft-versus-host disease. Transplantation 1988; 46: 402.

5. Dilly S, Sloane JP. Changes in rectal leucocytes after allogeneic bone marrow transplantation. Clin Exp Immunol 1987; 67: 151.

6. Norton J, Sloane JP, Al-Saffar N, Haskard DO. Vessel associated adhesion molecules in normal skin and acute graft-versus-host disease. J Clin Pathol 1991; 44: 586.

7. Davis R, Smoller BR. T lymphocytes expressing HECA-452 epitope are present in cutaneous acute graft-versus-host disease and erythema multiforme, but not in acute graft-versus-host disease in gut organs. Am J Pathol 1992; 141: 691.

8. Vie H, Millpied N, Devilder MC et al. Characterization of skin-infiltrating T lymphocytes during acute graft-versus-host disease. Hum Immunol 1990; 29: 110.

9. Acevedo A, Aramburu J, Lopez J et al. Identification of natural killer (NK) cells in lesions of human cutaneous graft-versus-host disease: Expression of a novel NK-associated surface antigen (Kp43) in mononuclear infiltrates. J Invest Dermatol 1991; 97: 659.

10. Ferrara J, Guillen FJ,van Dijken PJ, Marion A, Murphy GF, Burakoff SJ. Evidence that large granular lymphocyte of donor origin mediate acute graft-versus-host disease. Transplantation 1989; 47: 50.

11. Woodruff J, Hansen JA, Good RA, Santos GW, Slavin RE. The pathology of graft-versus-host reaction (GVHR) in adults receiving bone marrow transplants. Transpl Proc 1976; 8: 675.

12. Glucksberg H, Storb R, Fefer A et al. Clinical manifestations of graft-versus-host disease in human recipients of marrow from HLA-matched sibling donors. Transplantation 1974; 18: 295.

13. Norton J, Sloane JP, Al-Saffar N, Haskard DO. Expression of adhesion molecules in human intestinal graft-versus-host disease. Clin Exp Immunol 1992; 87: 231.

14. Garside P, Hutton AK, Severn A, Liew FY, Mowat AMI. Nitric oxide mediates intestimal pathology in graft-versus-host disease. Eur J Immunol 1992; 22: 2141.

15. Weisdorf D, Snover DC, Haake R. Acute upper gastrointestinal graft-versus-host disease: Clinical significance and response to immunosuppressive therapy. Blood 1990; 76: 624.

16. Iwasaki T, Fujiwara H, Shearer GM. Loss of proliferative capacity and T cell immune development potential of bone marrow from mice undergoing a graft-versus-host reaction. J Immunol 1986; 137: 3100.

17. Englehard D, Handsher R, Naparstek J, et al. Immune response to polio vaccination in bone marrow transplant recipients. Bone Marrow Transpl 1991 8: 295.

18. Vogelsang G, Hess AD, Santos GW. Acute graft-versus-host disease: Clinical characteristics in the cyclosporine era. Medicine 1988; 67: 163.

19. Vogelsang G, Wagner JE. Graft-versus-host disease. Hematol/Onc Clin NA 1990; 4: 625.

20. Atkinson K, Horowitz MM, Biggs JC, Gale RP, Rimm AA, Bortin MM. The clinical diagnosis of acute graft-versus-host disease: A diversity of views amongst marrow transplant centers. Bone Marrow Transpl 1988; 3: 5.

21. Portanova J, Ebling FM, Hammond WS, Hahn BH, Kotzin BL. Allogeneic MHC antigen requirements for lupus-like autoantibody production and nephritis in murine graft-versus-host disease. J Immunol 1988; 141: 3370.

22. Norhagen-Engstrom G, Hammarstrom L, Lonnqvist B, Soder P-O, Smith CIE. Ontogeny of immunoglobulins in bone marrow transplanted individuals: An analysis of serum and salivary levels. Transplantation 1988; 46: 710.

23. Elfenbein G, Anderson PN, Jumphrey RL et al. Immune system reconstitution following allogeneic bone marrow transplantation in man: A multiparameter analysis. Transplant Proc 1976; 8: 641.

24. Perreault C, Giasson M, Gyger M et al. Serum immunoglobulin levels following allogeneic bone marrow transplantation. Blut 1985; 51: 137.

25. Witherspoon R, Kopecky K, Storb, R et al. Immunological recovery in 48 patients following syngeneic marrow transplantation for hematological malignancy. Transplantation 1982; 33: 143.

26. Abedi MR, Hammarstrom L, Ringden O, Smith ECI. Development of IgA deficiency after bone marrow transplantation. Transplantation 1990; 50: 415.

27. Heyd J, Donnenburg AD, Burns WH, Saral R, Santos GW. Immunoglobin E levels following allogeneic, autologous and syngeneic bone marrow transplantation: An indirect asociation between hyperproduction and acute graft-versus-host disease in allogeneic BMT. Blood 1988; 72: 442.

28. Beatty P, Clift RA, Mickelson EM et al. Marrow transplantation from related donors other than HLA-identical siblings. N Engl J Med 1985; 313: 765.

29. Kato Y, Matsuishi Y, Cecka M et al. HLA-DP incompatibilities and severe graft-versus-host disease in unrelated bone marrow transplants. Transplantation 1991; 52: 374.

30. Weisdorf D, Hakke R, Blazar B et al. Risk factors for acute graft-versus-host disease in histocompatible donor bone marrow transplantation. Transplantation 1991; 51: 1197.

31. Nash R, Pepe MS, Storb R et al. Acute graft-versus-host disease: Analysis of risk factors after allogeneic marrow transplantation and prophylaxis with cyclosporine and methotrexate. Blood 1992; 80: 1838.

32. Bross D, Tutschka PJ, Farmer ER et al. Predictive factors for acute graft-versus-host disease in patients transplanted with HLA-identical bone marrow. Blood 1984; 63: 1265.

33. van Bekkum D, Roodenburg J, Heidt PJ, vander Waaij D. Mitigation of secondary disease of allogeneic mouse chimeras by modification of intestinal microflora. JNCI 1976; 52: 401.

34. Jones J, Wilson R, Bealmear PM. Mortality and gross pathology of secondary disease in germ-free mouse radiation chimeras. Radiat Res 1971; 45: 577.

35. Storb R, Prentice RL, Buckner CD et al. Graft-versus-host disease and survival in patients with aplastic anemia treated by marrow grafts from HLA-identical siblings. Beneficial effect of a protective enviroment. New Engl J Med 1983; 308: 302.

36. Beelen D, Haralambie E, Brandt H et al. Evidence that sustained growth suppression of intestinal anaerobic bacteria reduces the risk of acute graft-versus-host disease after sibling marrow transplantation. Blood 1992; 80: 2668.

37. van Bekkum D, Knaan S. Role of bacterial flora in the development of intestinal lesions from graft-versus-host reaction. J Natl Cancer Inst 1977; 58: 787.

38. Vossen J, Heidt PJ, van den Berg H, Gerritsen EJA, Hermans J, Dooren LJ. Prevention of infection and graft-versus-host disease by suppression of intestinal microflora in children treated with allogeneic bone marrow transplantation. Eur J Clin Micro Inf 1990; 9: 14.

39. Storb R, Prentice R, Hansen JA, Thomas ED. Association between HLA-B antigens and acute graft-versus-host disease. Lancet 1983; 2: 816.

40. Smyth L, Herrmann RP, Christiansen FT, Witt CS, Townend DC, Dawkins RL. Genetic factors influence the development of acute graft-versus-host disease in adults undergoing allogeneic bone marrow transplantation. Transpl Proc 1992; 24: 2269.

41. Holmes J, Whittaker JA. Histocompatibility antigen DR4 is associated with chronic graft-versus-host disease in the South Wales population. Br J Haematol 1989; 73: 424.

42. Yee G, Slef SG, McGuire TR, Carlin JC, Sanders JE, Deeg HJ. Serum cyclosporine concentration and risk of acute graft-versus-host disease after allogeneic marrow transplantation. N Engl J Med 1988; 319: 65.

43. Michallet M, Corront B, Bosson JL et al. Role of splenectomy in incidence and severity of acute graft-versus-host disease: A multicenter study of 157 patients. Bone Marrow Transpl 1991; 8: 13.

44. Gratama J, Nat HVD, Weiland HT et al. Intensification of GVHD prophylaxis interferes with the effects of pretransplant herpes virus serology on the occurrence of grades II-IV acute graft-versus-host disease. Ann Hematol 1992; 64: A137.

45. Widmer M, Bach FH. Antigen-driven helper cell independent cloned cytolytic T lymphocytes. Nature 1981; 294: 750.

46. Gutterman J, Rossen RD, Butler WT et al. Immunoglobulin on tumor cells and tumor-induced lymphocyte blastogenesis in human acute leukemia. N Engl J Med 1973; 288: 169.

47. Fefer A, Mickelson E, Thomas ED. Leukaemia antigens: Stimulation of lymphocytes in mixed culture by cells from HLA identical siblings. Clin Exp Immunol 1976; 23: 214.

48. Rudolph R, Mickelson E, Thomas ED. Mixed leukocyte reactivity and leukemia: Study of identical siblings. J Clin Invest 1970; 49: 2271.

49. Fridman W, Kourilsky FM. Stimulation of lymphocytes by autologous leukemia cells in acute leukemia. Nature 1969; 224: 277.

50. Bach M, Bach FH, Joo P. Leukemia-associated antigens in the mixed leucocyte culture test. Science 1969; 166: 1520.

51. Pawelec , Muller C, Ehninger G. Predictive strength of mixed lymphocyte cultures for acute graft-verus-host disease in patients transplanted with HLA-identical sibling bone marrow. Transplantation 1989; 48: 890.

52. Sondel P, Hank JA, Wendel T, Flynn B, Bordeck MH. HLA identical leukemic cells and T cell growth factor activate cytotoxic T cell recognition of minor histocompatibility antigens in vitro. J Clin Invest 1983; 71: 1779.

53. Johnsen H, Bostrom L, Moller J, Jorgensen JA, Jensen L, Ringden O. A study of donor alloreactivity, which may predict acute graft-versus-host disease in HLA identical bone marrow transplantations for early leukemia. Scand J Immunol 1992; 35: 353.

54. Johnsen H, Mickelson E, Beatty PG, Hansen JA. Donor alloreactivity may predict acute graft-versus host disease in patients receiving marrow transplants from HLA identical siblings. Bone Marrow Transpl 1992; 9: 91.

55. Vogelsang G, Hess AD, Berkman A et al. An in vitro predictive test for graft-versus-host disease in patients with genotypic HLA-identical bone marrow transplants. N Engl J Med 1985; 313: 645.

56. Dickinson A, Sviland L, Carey P et al. Skin explant culture as a model for cutaneous graft-versus-host disease in humans. Bone Marrow Transpl 1988; 3: 323.

57. Bagot M, Cordonnier C, Tilkin AF et al. A possible predictive test for graft-versus-host disease in bone marrow graft recipients: The mixed epidermal cell-lymphocyte reaction. Transplantation 1986. 41: p. 316-319.

58. Bagot M, Mary J-Y, Heslan M et al. The mixed epidermal cell lymphocyte-reaction is the most predictive factor of acute graft-versus-host disease in bone marrow graft recipients. Br J Haematol 1988; 70: 403.

59. Rosenstein Y, Ratnofsky S, Burakoff SJ, Herrmann SH. Direct evidence for binding of CD8 to HLA class I antigens. J Exp Med 1989; 169: 149.

60. Westhoff U, Doxiadis I, Beelen D, Schaefer U, Grosse-Wilde H. Soluble HLA class I concentrations and GVHD after allogeneic marrow transplantation. Transplantation 1989; 48: 891.

61. Thompson S, Wareham M, Pearson ADJ, Sviland L, Turner GA. A preliminary study of serum class II levels in healthy individuals and bone marrow transplant patients. Clin Chim Acta 1989; 185: 45.

# CHAPTER 8

# Clinical Trials

Clinically significant acute GVHD occurs in 9-50% of patients who receive an allogeneic bone marrow graft from a genotypically HLA identical sibling, even though these patients receive intensive prophylaxis with immunosuppressive agents such as methotrexate, cyclosporine, corticosteroids or anti-thymocyte globulin. Development of moderate (grade II) or severe (grade III or IV) acute GVHD after marrow transplantation is associated with a significant decrease in survival. Various methods to prevent GVHD have been developed. The mainstay of prophylaxis remains pharmacological combination of drugs which individually have been shown to prevent GVHD.

## DRUG PROPHYLAXIS

As with any disease, effective prevention is, by far, one of the more important aspects of GVHD. Prevention of GVHD for improved outcome following allogeneic marrow grafting has been sought since the first human allogeneic bone marrow transplants were complicated by GVHD (Table 8.1). However, three small trials have been reported where no GVHD

*Table 8.1. Drug prophylaxis for GVHD*

| Drug(s) | GVHD | Improved disease-free survival | Ref. |
|---|---|---|---|
| None | 52-100% | – | 1, 2, 3 |
| Cyclophosphamide | 55% | – | 6 |
| Methotrexate | 56-70% | – | 5, 7 |
| Anti–thymocyte globulin/methotrexate | 21% | – | 11 |
| Cyclosporine | 33-54% |  | 15, 16, 17 |
| Cyclosporine/Methotrexate | 15-33% | no | 22-28 |
| Cyclosporine/Prednisone | 12-21% | no | 32, 33, 34, 38 |
| Cyclosporine/Methotrexate/Prednisone | 9-32% | no | 33, 39, 41 |

prophylaxis was used.[1,2] The results of these trials did not demonstrate any difference in overall survival or in the incidence of chronic GVHD (although there may be a difference in the severity of chronic GVHD). There were differences among these studies. In the Seattle trial, where no prophylaxis was used in 15 evaluable patients, 100% of the patients had grade II or greater graft-versus-host disease.[1] In the second study, 67% of the patients developed GVHD if no postgrafting prophylaxis was used compared to 25-26%, if methotrexate or methotrexate and prednisone were used, but there was no difference in survival.[3] However, this was a small study with only 15 patients not receiving any prophylaxis. Both of these studies suggested a higher incidence of acute GVHD when no postgrafting prophylaxis was used. The results were different in another nonrandomized study where no postgrafting GVHD prophylaxis was administered.[2] Among the 34 patients given methotrexate for prophylaxis of GVHD, 59% developed GVHD compared to 52% of patients who did not receive any prophylaxis. The reason for such differences may be due to patient selection and the overall small numbers of patients studied. There is no doubt, however, that the occurrence of GVHD can have a devastating effect on patients and subsequent studies have shown that there is an impact in overall survival. Given the advances in GVHD prophylaxis to date, it is unlikely that clinical investigators would consider not using any GVHD prophylaxis following unmanipulated bone marrow grafts.

## SINGLE AGENTS

Various methods to prevent the occurrence of GVHD have been devised over the years. The initial studies used a single drug for the prophylaxis of GVHD. As mentioned earlier, studies by Uphoff demonstrated that the use of aminopterin in mice receiving allogeneic BMT decreased the incidence of GVHD.[4] Similar results were seen in dogs, where the use of methotrexate resulted in a greater than 90% disease-free survival following BMT from DLA identical litter mates compared to a 55% incidence of acute GVHD and only a 45% survival in those dogs not receiving any GVHD prophylaxis.[5] In 1966, Santos and Owens described the use of cyclophosphamide and demonstrated that it was useful for the prevention and treatment of GVHD in rats.[6] Yet, despite the use of single drug prophylaxis, GVHD still occurred in up to 55-70% of patients.[7,8] Until the introduction of cyclosporine, these two drugs served as the mainstay of therapy.

## ANTI-THYMOCYTE GLOBULIN

Anti-thymocyte globulin (ATG) has also been used. Two studies compared the addition of ATG to methotrexate and did not find a decrease in the incidence of GVHD.[9,10] A third study from the BMT group in Minnesota found that when ATG was combined with methotrexate and prednisone there was a decrease of acute GVHD from 48% to 21%.[11] The addition of anti-thymocyte globulin appeared to improve the incidence of GVHD, however, there was no difference in survival.

## CYCLOSPORINE

Cyclosporine A was introduced in the 1970's. The mechanism of its action is related to its ability to bind to cyclophilin, a cytosolic transporter protein. The drug is then carried into the nucleus where it can bind to the IL-2 promoter region, preventing IL-2 gene expression and activation of T lymphocytes. Tolerance is induced with inhibition of cytotoxic T cells and with relative sparing of antigen-specific T cells. Animal studies demonstrated that cyclosporine was a potent agent to prevent GVHD.[12] Early uncontrolled trials also demonstrated the usefulness of cyclosporine in reducing the incidence of GVHD and improving survival.[13,14] For the purposes of most trials, prevention of GVHD is measured primarily on the prevention of significant GVHD, that is grade II or greater. Grade I GVHD does not carry a clinically adverse outcome unless it progresses to more extensive GVHD. All of these and subsequent studies discussed will be primarily matched related BMT.

Controlled follow-up studies of cyclosporine showed that although it is a useful agent, cyclosporine was not superior to methotrexate or cyclophosphamide.[7,15,16] A study of 75 patients, in which 33% of the patients on cyclosporine and 56% on methotrexate developed acute GVHD of grade II-IV, nearly reached statistical significance (p=0.07). Recent follow-up of three of these studies (179 patients) compared cyclosporine versus methotrexate with follow-up ranging from 8 to 11 years. The long term follow up also allowed for analysis of disease-free survival as well as of leukemic relapse.[17] Although patients with advanced disease receiving cyclosporine had a trend towards higher relapse rates, this difference did not reach statistical significance. Relapse rates were identical for all three groups (advanced hematological malignancy, acute myelogenous leukemia in first complete remission and chronic myelogenous leukemia). Not only was there no difference in their ability to prevent GVHD, but these two drugs were associated with similar incidence of interstitial pneumonitis. Others suggest, however, that there may be an increased risk of relapse for those treated with cyclosporine (42%) compared to methotrexate (10%). The total number of patients included in this study was only 59.[18]

Another approach has been a prolonged course of GVHD prophylaxis with cyclosporine and early treatment of acute GVHD with high-dose corticosteroids.[19] Under this regimen, cyclosporine was tapered very slowly after 12 months. Acute GVHD was treated at the first clear sign of the disease with methylprednisolone at 10-20 mg/kg/day divided into four doses. This regimen proved to be quite efficacious for GVHD. Unfortunately, the total number of patients was relatively small (45 patients). Nonetheless, the investigators observed the low incidence of severe GVHD (5%) and of chronic GVHD (9%). This is a potential approach for an effective therapy with decreased morbidity associated with prolonged corticosteroid use.

## COMBINATION PROPHYLAXIS

The initial comparison studies of single agents in the prophylaxis of GVHD did not show significant differences. These results led to renewed interest in the combination of cyclosporine and methotrexate for GVHD prophylaxis. Studies in dogs that received DLA-nonidentical marrow from unrelated dogs and DLA-haploidentical marrow from litter mates, demonstrated a significant reduction in the incidence of acute GVHD and an improvement in survival in favor of those receiving cyclosporine and a short course of methotrexate.[20,21] Several clinical trials, carried out in Seattle and elsewhere, have shown a survival advantage for patients who received the combination of cyclosporine and methotrexate compared to either one of those drugs utilized alone.[22,23] A large retrospective study of 595 patients with aplastic anemia receiving allogeneic bone marrow transplants analyzed the effect of three GVHD regimens: methotrexate, cyclosporine and methotrexate plus cyclosporine.[24] Patients who received cyclosporine with or without methotrexate had a significantly higher probability of five-year survival (69%) compared to patients receiving methotrexate only (56%). The higher survival rate with cyclosporine was related to a lower incidence of interstitial pneumonia and chronic GVHD.

Two prospective randomized trials in patients with leukemia or aplastic anemia have shown that the combination of cyclosporine and methotrexate was superior to either drug alone in preventing GVHD.[25,26] The first trial treated 93 patients with acute myelogenous leukemia in first complete remission or chronic myelogenous leukemia in chronic phase.[26] The patients randomized to receive the combination of cyclosporine and methotrexate had a 33% cumulative incidence of developing acute GVHD compared to 54% for the patients receiving cyclosporine alone. The second trial compared the same combination of cyclosporine and methotrexate to methotrexate alone, again showing a superior advantage in favor of the combination of drugs. Another trial investigated the use of this combination regimen of cyclosporine and methotrexate in patients with leukemia and aplastic anemia.[27] The cumulative incidence of acute GVHD in patients with leukemia was approximately 32% for those receiving the combination compared to 55% for those receiving cyclosporine alone. For patients with aplastic anemia, the combination of drug resulted in only 18% grade II-IV acute GVHD compared to 52% for those receiving cyclosporine alone. The long-term follow up results of these trials were reported recently.[17,28] In the most recent analyses of patients treated with the combination of cyclosporine and methotrexate, there was a significant decrease in the incidence and severity of acute GVHD. In this trial none of the patients receiving the combination chemoprophylaxis developed grade IV GVHD. There was no effect on the rate of development of chronic GVHD. There was a trend towards improved event-free survival in the subgroup of patients with chronic myelogenous leukemia. However, in patients with acute myelogenous leukemia, the early survival benefit was offset by an increase in the relapse rate.

A comparison of three regimens: cyclosporine alone, T-cell depletion, and the combination of cyclosporine and methotrexate was studied in 140 consecutive patients with chronic myelogenous leukemia.[29] The results suggest that the combination of cyclosporine and methotrexate is the best of the three options for improved disease-free survival. Presently, the combination of cyclosporine and methotrexate is the most widely used regimen for the prophylaxis of acute GVHD.

Various modifications of the basic regimen developed in Seattle have been investigated. None of these studies have compared the changes to the standard cyclosporine and methotrexate in a prospective randomized fashion. One study used six weeks of continuous intravenous cyclosporine rather than switching to oral administration. This regimen included a short course of methotrexate. Cyclosporine was continued intravenously until day +45 and switched to oral cyclosporine until day +90 after which it was discontinued. The regimen was well-tolerated and resulted in only 16% acute GVHD and in only 13% de novo chronic GVHD.[30] A recent pilot study from the same group suggests that perhaps a slight modification in the dosing of cyclosporine may reduce toxicity while maintaining efficacy.[31] Nineteen patients received a 50% decrease in the dose of cyclosporine for the first two weeks. When the results of this pilot study was compared to a matched cohort, there was no difference in the incidence of acute GVHD (42% versus 51% in the standard dose group). However, patients receiving the "low-dose" prophylaxis appeared to have less hepatotoxicity and the prescribed doses of methotrexate and cyclosporine were administered closer to the intended doses. Use of this regimen, however, still resulted in an incidence of acute GVHD (grade II-IV) of 20-30%.[26,28]

While prednisone is the most effective drug in the therapy of acute GVHD, its use in combination with cyclosporine, methotrexate, or cyclophosphamide is effective for prophylaxis of acute GVHD.[8,11,32-36] This regimen of cyclosporine and prednisone was compared to the regimen of cyclosporine and methotrexate as developed in Seattle in a multi-institution trial.[37] The primary purpose of this study was to evaluate the preparatory regimen consisting of busulfan and cyclophosphamide in patients with chronic myelogenous leukemia. Patients were not randomized to the two GVHD regimens. The results demonstrated that the incidence of GVHD was 29% for those receiving cyclosporine and prednisone compared to 38% for those receiving cyclosporine and methotrexate (p=NS). It is likely that the choice of GVHD prophylactic regimen was dependent on the institution where the BMT occurred.

In 1976, City of Hope investigators designed and implemented a series of sequential trials for the prophylaxis of acute GVHD. In a prospective randomized study comparing methotrexate and prednisone to cyclosporine, the investigators observed a reduction of grade II-IV acute GVHD from 47 to 28% with the cyclosporine and prednisone combination.[32] In 1986, they modified the combination of cyclosporine and prednisone by increasing the dose of prednisone and starting it on day +7, as described by the Ohio State group, rather than day +15.[35] This change was tested in a phase II trial resulting in an incidence of grade II-IV acute GVHD of 12% (S. Forman, unpublished). Subsequently, the BMT groups at the City of Hope and Stanford University conducted a randomized study to determine if the addition of three doses of methotrexate to the combination of cyclosporine and prednisone (as used in the 1986 phase II trial) could further decrease the incidence of acute GVHD. This attempted to improve the prophylaxis of acute GVHD by the addition of three doses of methotrexate to the cyclosporine and prednisone regimen. The rationale for using only three doses of methotrexate was two-fold: first, a large number of patients never receive the fourth dose of methotrexate because of cumulative toxicity, and second, out of concern for the potential added toxicity of this GVHD regimen to the preparatory regimen containing etoposide. This study was a prospective randomized trial evaluating acute GVHD in two groups that were well-balanced in terms of the characteristics typically associated with the occurrence of acute GVHD.

During the five-year period between December 1986 and December 1991, 150 patients participated in the study.[33] These patients represented a uniform group of "best risk candidates" with either acute leukemia, lymphoblastic leukemia in first remission, or chronic myelogenous leukemia in first chronic phase. Patients with acute lymphoblastic leukemia or lymphoma were considered to be "high risk" for relapse. All patients received their marrow grafts from genotypically matched donors. Patients were stratified in the randomization by age and type of leukemia. One hundred forty-nine patients were evaluable for analysis. One patient died on day 19 (after transplantation and prior to engraftment) and was not evaluable for GVHD, but was included in the survival analysis. All other patients survived for at least 32 days after marrow grafting. Three patients were randomized but refused to receive the assigned treatment combination; two patients were randomized to cyclosporine, methotrexate and prednisone but chose to receive the two-drug arm, while one patient, randomized to cyclosporine and prednisone, preferred to receive the three-drug combination. One additional patient was randomized to the three-drug arm, but developed renal insufficiency and never received any methotrexate. All 149 patients evaluable for GVHD were analyzed as they were originally randomized (intent-to-treat analysis). All patients received a uniform preparatory regimen consisting of total body irradiation, 1320 cGy, in 11 fractions on day -7 through day -4, and 60 mg/kg of etoposide intravenously over four hours on day -3. The bone marrow was infused on day 0.

All patients received cyclosporine by continuous intravenous infusion as a loading dose starting on day -2. Figure 8.1 illustrates the dosing schema. Serum cyclosporine levels were measured twice a week using an immunoassay

| Day | Cyclosporine | Prednisone | Methotrexate |
|-----|-------------|------------|--------------|
| -2 | 5.0 mg/kg IV daily | – | |
| +1 | " | – | 15 mg/m$^2$ IV single dose |
| +3 | " | – | 10 mg/m$^2$ IV single dose |
| +4 | 3.0 mg/kg IV daily | – | |
| +6 | " | – | 10 mg/m$^2$ IV single dose |
| +7 | " | 0.5 mg/kg IV daily | |
| | " | " | |
| +15 | 3.75 mg/kg IV daily | 1.0 mg/kg IV daily | |
| | " | " | |
| +29 | " | 0.8 mg/kg PO daily | |
| +36 | 10 mg/kg PO daily | " | |
| +43 | " | 0.5 mg/kg PO daily | |
| | " | " | |
| +57 | " | 0.2 mg/kg PO daily | |
| +84 | 8 mg/kg PO daily | " | |
| | " | " | |
| +98 | 6 mg/kg PO daily | " | |
| | " | " | |
| +120 | 4 mg/kg PO daily | 0.1 mg/kg PO daily | |
| | " | " | |
| +180 | off | off | |

Fig. 8.1. Schema for the triple drug prophylaxis.

(TDx System, Abbott Laboratories, Abbott Park, IL). For those patients randomized to receive methotrexate, the dose was reduced using a sliding scale if significant renal or hepatic dysfunction was present or if mucositis was extensive. Methylprednisolone was increased to 2 mg/kg daily if grade II-IV acute GVHD occurred.

In this study, methylprednisolone was begun on day +7 rather than on day +15, and the dose of methylprednisolone used was higher than in the previous trials. The dose of cyclosporine and prednisone regimen was identical to that reported by the Ohio State University group. The results of the phase III study using cyclosporine and prednisone were not as good as those obtained in the earlier phase II trial. However, the new data corroborated the results obtained in other studies of prophylaxis of acute GVHD with cyclosporine and prednisone, including a recently completed Southwest Oncology Group trial.[38]

As demonstrated in Figure 8.2, patients receiving cyclosporine, methotrexate and prednisone had a significantly lower incidence of grade II-IV acute GVHD (9%) compared to those receiving cyclosporine and prednisone (23%, p=0.02). Multivariate Cox regression analysis demonstrated an

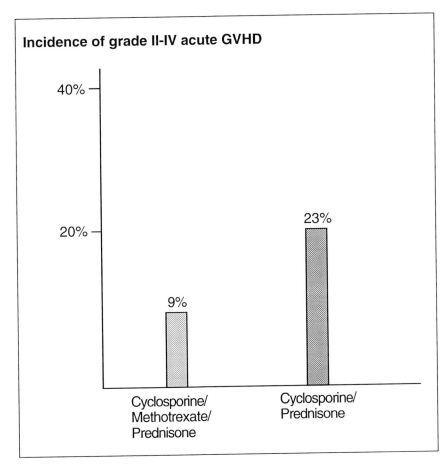

*Fig. 8.2. Incidence of grade II-IV acute GVHD comparing cyclosporine, methotrexate and prednisone to cyclosporine and prednisone for the prophylaxis of GVHD.*

increased risk of acute GVHD associated with an elevated creatinine (p=0.006) and randomization to cyclosporine and prednisone (p=0.02). This lower incidence of acute GVHD did not result in a higher relapse rate. There was no statistically significant difference in disease-free survival at three years between the two treatment arms (64% for the triple drug regimen versus 59% for the two-drug combination, p=0.57).

The cumulative incidence and characteristics of chronic GVHD are similar to those described by others.[7,8,39] More importantly, very few patients were affected significantly by chronic GVHD. Most patients had mild skin or buccal mucosal changes that did not affect their daily activities. However, eight patients died of chronic GVHD-associated infections or bronchiolitis obliterans in the treatment group receiving cyclosporine and prednisone while three patients died of chronic GVHD in the treatment group receiving cyclosporine, methotrexate and prednisone. The median Karnofsky performance status was 90% in both groups and, as described previously, the majority of patients in this trial enjoy a good quality of life.[40]

Although there was a statistically significant decrease in the occurrence of grade II-IV acute GVHD in the group of patients receiving methotrexate, no difference in disease-free survival was noted. This study was designed to investigate only a short-term goal, the occurrence of acute GVHD. In addition, because the number of each adverse event was low in the two groups, a small difference in causes for failure was unlikely to affect overall disease-free survival outcome. The two late deaths in the group receiving the three drug arm were secondary to relapse in one patient and bronchiolitis obliterans in another patient. Therefore, because both groups of patients fared relatively well with three-year, disease-free survival rates of 59% and 64%, enrollment of a considerably larger number of patients would be required to detect a significant difference in disease-free survival.

A previous study from Seattle using the addition of prednisone to cyclosporine and methotrexate did not demonstrate an advantage of this three-drug regimen.[39] The investigators found a higher incidence of acute GVHD in the patients receiving cyclosporine, prednisone and methotrexate when high dose prednisone (2 mg/kg) was begun on day +1 after allografting. In the same study, if prednisone began on day +15, there was no difference in the incidence of acute GVHD compared to patients not receiving prednisone. While this study from Seattle appears similar to our study, the dose schedules of prednisone and methotrexate are different. Our schedule of methotrexate consisted of three rather than four doses, given before prednisone treatment was initiated. This difference in sequence of methotrexate and prednisone may explain the difference in the incidence of grade II-IV acute GVHD that we observed as compared to the Seattle study. Initiation of prednisone after all doses of methotrexate were delivered would not be expected to interfere with the cytolytic action of methotrexate on donor lymphocytes that proliferate in response to host alloantigens. Beginning prednisone on day +7 may be early enough to eliminate or inhibit residual lymphocytes (host or donor) that are important in the afferent arm of acute GVHD.

A second randomized study compared prospectively the combination of cyclosporine and methotrexate to cyclosporine, methotrexate and prednisolone for prevention of GVHD.[41] In this study of 41 patients, there were no differences between the two arms for the incidence of acute GVHD, chronic GVHD, interstitial pneumonitis, relapse, survival and disease-free survival. The actuarial incidence for the two-drug regimen was 15% compared to 10% for the three-drug regimen (p=NS). Leukemic relapse was the principal cause of failure in this study. However, the prednisolone was also begun on day 0 and the cyclosporine and methotrexate doses were lower than those used in our or the Seattle studies.

Finally, we selected a uniform patient population of "best risk" candidates for allogeneic BMT. We believe this to be the ideal group to study the question of acute GVHD prophylaxis because it minimizes the confounding factors of variable preparatory regimens and differences in disease status. This ideal patient population may also explain in part the lower incidence of acute GVHD and our low incidence of disease recurrence.[42] Our study did not address the question of whether the addition of prednisone to the most widely used regimen of cyclosporine and methotrexate (developed in Seattle) resulted in a lower incidence of acute GVHD. Rather, it was designed to explore whether the combination of cyclosporine, methotrexate and prednisone given in the manner described was superior to our previous regimen of cyclosporine and prednisone. Use of the three-drug regimen resulted in a low incidence of grade II-IV acute GVHD of 9% and was statistically superior when compared to cyclosporine and prednisone. Continued experience with this regimen in patients with more partially matched related donors or in matched unrelated donor marrow transplantation will further define the role of this three-drug regimen for the prevention of acute GVHD.

Studies have compared combination prophylaxis of cyclosporine and methotrexate to T-cell depletion.[43] Unfortunately, the total number of patients per arm was relatively small. The results of this trial support data presented earlier suggesting that patients who were randomized to methotrexate alone had a decreased risk of relapse compared to those treated with cyclosporine. There was no difference in outcome for those patients treated with cyclosporine and methotrexate compared to those receiving T cell-depleted marrow grafts.

A concern about the use of combination regimens, and specifically methotrexate, is hepatotoxicity. One study found a marked increase in the hepatotoxicity in patients who received cyclosporine and methotrexate for graft-versus-host disease prophylaxis and the preparative regimen consisting of busulfan and cyclophosphamide.[44] There was an increase in veno-occlusive disease (VOD) from 18-70% and the death rate caused by VOD increased from 4.5% to 25% compared to patients who received cyclosporine and prednisone for GVHD prophylaxis. This study suggested the relative toxicity of combining methotrexate and busulfan.

Clinical correlation with cyclosporine blood levels has been attempted. The results of four different methods of GVHD prophylaxis in a single institution compared methotrexate, cyclosporine, methotrexate and cyclosporine, and T cell-depletion and cyclosporine. Using four different assays for measurement of cyclosporine blood levels, no correlation was detected by any method that correlated with the clinical outcome.[45] Another study attempted to monitor the therapeutic levels of cyclosporine when used with methotrexate. This resulted in a 60% reduction of cyclosporine dosage by day +50 compared to the Seattle protocol. This apparently did not result in an increased incidence of acute GVHD or a higher relapse rate.[46]

## ANTIBODIES

Anti-thymocyte globulin (ATG) has been given for prophylaxis of GVHD, as GVHD is caused by donor T lymphocytes.[47] The results of this trial were not as encouraging to warrant its use as a first line therapy. Since T cells become activated by histocompatibility antigens that differ between host and donor, there is an increase in the expression of IL-2 receptors. The IL-2 receptor is composed of at least two chains, a heavy chain (75 kd) and a light chain (55 kd) that combine to form a molecular complex with high affinity to IL-2.[48] The binding of IL-2 to its receptor is an essential requirement for T-cell proliferation. Murine monoclonal antibodies that can bind to a human IL-2 receptor light chain and block the IL-2 binding have been used to treat and as prophylaxis against GVHD.[49] These IL-2 receptor-specific monoclonal antibodies may also allow selective targeting and destruction of activated T cells. A murine monoclonal IgG1 antibody (2A3), targeting specifically the 55 kd chain of the human IL-2 receptor was used as prophylaxis for acute GVHD. Eleven patients received both cyclosporine and methotrexate as used standardly in conjunction with antibody 2A3, 1 mg/kg on day -1, and .5 mg/kg daily from day 0 through day 19. There was no appreciable toxicity or adverse effect on engraftment. Seventy percent of patients, however, developed grade II-IV acute GVHD. These results suggest that administration of this particular antibody suppressed and delayed the activation of alloantigen-specific T cells but did not result in the elimination of these cells and, therefore, did not have a significant impact in the prophylaxis of GVHD. Newer agents directed against human IL-2 receptors may be more immunosuppressive and more efficacious.

Another anti-IL-2 receptor monoclonal antibody (33B3.1) was also used in the prevention of acute GVHD in 15 patients.[50] There were no major adverse clinical experiences noted. No GVHD occurred while the antibody was administered, although these patients also received a short course of methotrexate and cyclosporine A postgraft immunosuppression. These preliminary data suggest that a larger trial may show the efficacy of such an approach in the prophylaxis of acute GVHD.

Another approach has been the use of monoclonal antibodies targeted against various adhesion molecules. The ICAM-1/LFA-1 cell adhesion pathway is the critical pathway for the regulation of various immune functions including T-cell proliferation response to antigen, as well as T-cell and NK-cell cytotoxicity.[51,52] In a murine model of acute lethal GVHD treatment of host mice with either anti-LFA-1 or the mouse homologue of ICAM-1 (MLA2) resulted in a significantly decreased incidence of GVHD with enhanced survival.[53] Such an approach clearly could improve the outcome of allogeneic transplantation by decreasing GVHD.

Other monoclonal antibodies (anti-I-A, anti-L3T4 and anti-LFA-1) have been administered in monitoring the development of a murine cutaneous GVHD. Local administration of either anti-LyT4 or LFA-1, but not with anti-I-A, resulted in prevention of cutaneous GVHD. This would suggest that an I-A antigen-independent mechanism may also be operative in the development of cutaneous GVHD. The anti-LFA-1 monoclonal antibody appeared to be the most pertinent in inhibiting cutaneous GVHD, suggesting that LFA-1 may be involved in the epidermal invasion of T cells. The antibody appeared to function even if it was used after the establishment of cutaneous GVHD.

We also tested monoclonal antibodies against selected adhesion receptors of the immunoglobulin superfamily (ICAM-1, VCAM-1) and of the integrins (LFA-1, VLA-4) in an MLR across major MHC barriers, in secondary MLR across minor histocompatibility antigens, in a CD4$^+$ mediated hybridoma T-cell response, and in a CD8$^+$-mediated primed CTL response against minor histocompatibility antigens.[54] The results of these in vitro studies suggest that the overall effect was in the following direction: ICAM1 > LFA-1 > VCAM-1 > VLA-4. We also tested these monoclonal antibodies in a murine model of BMT across minor histocompatibility complex differences (B10.D2 → Balb/c) in an in vivo model. Treatment with anti-VLA-4 delayed the onset of GVHD, but failed to reduce the incidence, severity or GVHD-related mortality. In marked contrast, anti-VCAM-1 treatment reduced the incidence of GVHD on day 70 from 100% in controls to 55.6% (p<0.05) and significantly decreased GVHD-related mortality.

### Intravenous Immunoglobulins

Following marrow transplantation, serum Ig levels decrease dramatically. Under normal circumstances, IgG and IgM return to normal at approximately three to four months following allogeneic transplantation. Serum IgA levels may remain low for up to two years. Other studies have reported subclass deficiencies of IgG2 and IgG4 even though total normal serum IgG levels are normal.[55,56] Initial studies of intravenous immunoglobulins (IVIg) following BMT were to achieve a reduction of incidence and severity of cytomegalovirus (CMV) infections. However, in a large randomized study by Sullivan et al there was a reduced incidence of gram-negative septicemia and local infections in patients receiving IVIg, as well as a reduced incidence of acute GVHD in patients aged 20 years and older who received IVIg compared to the randomized control patients.[57] The data, therefore, demonstrated that the role of IVIg results in an immunomodulatory effect specifically in preventing GVHD.

## T-CELL DEPLETION

One attractive approach to prevent GVHD is to eliminate T lymphocytes from the donor inoculum prior to infusion of the bone marrow. This technique is effective in preventing acute GVHD across both major and minor histocompatibility barriers in mice. These early data in animal models led to many clinical trials in patients receiving bone marrow transplantation for leukemias. Several techniques have been developed to deplete T lymphocytes from donor bone marrow in humans including a variety of physical separation techniques such as density gradients, selective depletion with lectins, treatment with cytotoxic drugs, and the use of anti-T-cell serum or monoclonal antibodies, either alone, with complement, or conjugated to toxins. The depletion of T lymphocytes from donor bone marrow may also have adverse effects. T-cell depletion adversely affects engraftment, the adequacy of immune reconstitution, and the incidence of leukemic relapse or infections. Table 8.2 summarizes the current data of T-cell depletion.

*Table 8.2. T-cell depletion studies*

| n | Antibody prophylaxis | Other | GVHD | Relapse | Graft failure | Ref. |
|---|---|---|---|---|---|---|
| 20 | 8 monoclonals | cyclosporine/ methotrexate | 15% | 35% | 15% | 67 |
| 20 | anti-CD2 | cyclosporine | 15% | 25% | 60% | 59 |
| 58 | anti-CD2,5,7 or anti-CD4,5,8 | none | 5% | 24% | 19% | 68 |
| 36 | anti-CD8 | cyclosporine | 28% | 8% | 11% | 66 |
| 282 | Campath-1 | – | 12% | – | 15% | 62 |
| 112 | anti-CD6 | none | 6.2% | – | 2.7% | 73 |
| 122 | SBA/E–rosette | none | 6.4% | – | 16% | 77 |

Several techniques for T-cell depletion have been utilized. Most of these use ex vivo treatment of the donor bone marrow with monoclonal antibodies. The most common methods include broadly reactive anti-T-cell agents, such as anti-CD2, anti-CD3, anti-CD5, as well as those with more restricted reactivity such as anti-CD8 monoclonal antibodies.[58-61] A broadly reactive human monoclonal against lymphoid tissues, Campath-1 has also been used.[62] The first human trials involved simply the addition of the monoclonal antibody to the harvested bone marrow. It was hoped that antibody dependent cellular cytotoxicity, as well as human complement, would fix the antibody and cause cell lysis. These studies did not succeed.[58,60] Subsequent studies used ex vivo treatment with monoclonal antibodies with rabbit complement. Although these studies have shown some efficacy, the amount of variability between batches of complement and the different antibodies led to the development of newer methods of T-cell depletion. These include antibodies bound to ricin A chain, other toxins or antibodies conjugated to magnetic beads, depletion of an antibody bound to target cells, soybean lectin and agglutination and E-rosette formation or counterflow elutriation.[60,63,64] Most of these techniques generally achieve between a 1.5 to 4 log reduction of T cells. Unfortunately, most of these T-cell depletion methodologies result in either graft failure or a higher incidence of relapse and there is no significant overall improvement in disease-free survival.

Graft failure appears to occur in two general forms. The first form occurs when approximately half the patients have no signs of hematopoietic recovery. The second form occurs where there is delayed graft failure. These patients achieve an early engraftment with hematopoietic recovery, however, over several weeks to months, pancytopenia occurs again. The incidence of leukemic relapse has also been increased following transplantation in T cell-depleted marrow. The risk of relapse appears to be different for different leukemias. In a recent analysis from the International Bone Marrow Transplant Registry, patients with chronic myelogenous leukemia in chronic phase had a relapse rate of approximately 12% following unmodified bone marrow transplants. This risk increased to 50% in patients who received T-cell-depleted transplants.[65] High relapse rates are also seen in patients transplanted for acute nonlymphoblastic leukemia and acute lymphoblastic leukemia; however, the differences in these groups were not as dramatic.[66]

The initial studies of T-cell depletion were reported in the early 1980s. The Seattle group reported 20 patients treated with a panel of eight different monoclonal antibodies against T cells.[67] These patients all received prophylaxis with cyclosporine. The overall incidence of GVHD was 15%; however, graft failure was high at 20%. Relapse was also high, but this was not significantly different from their experience with the same type of patients using standard chemotherapy for prophylaxis. The results of the UCLA trial were also described.[59] Again, a total of 20 patients received a monoclonal antibody directed against CD2, a pan T-cell antigen. These patients also received prophylaxis with methotrexate and cyclosporine. The overall incidence of GVHD was low at 15% with a graft failure rate of 20%. However, both of these trials used chemical prophylaxis in addition to the T cell-depletion process. The relapse rate was high given that these were the best- to good-risk patients.

A third report was presented by the Groupe d'Étude de la Greffe de Moelle Osseuse (GEGMO).[68] This was a large group of 58 patients utilizing a panel of monoclonal antibodies directed against CD2, CD5 and CD7 versus CD4, CD5 and CD8. These patients received no other prophylaxis for graft-versus-host disease. The incidence of graft-versus-host disease was low at 5% with a graft failure rate not very different from the previous two studies. The overall relapse rate of 24% was not different from that reported for those patients prepared with total body irradiation and cyclophosphamide.

The largest study of T-cell depletion was with 282 leukemia patients with bone marrow transplantation from HLA-matched siblings using marrow depleted of T cells with Campath-1 and autologous complement. The incidence of grade II-IV GVHD was 12%. The incidence of graft failure was 15%. The major impact in relapse was in patients with chronic myelogenous leukemia.[62] In this study, the most important predictive factor for relapse appeared to be slow engraftment. Graft failure was almost certainly due to graft rejection by residual recipient T cells that survived the conditioning protocol. In a separate study using this same antibody, however, Campath-1 was given in vivo in an attempt to prevent GVHD rather than using it ex vivo to treat the bone marrow.[69] Twenty-two patients were treated. The patients received the standard preparative regimen of cyclophosphamide and a single dose of total body irradiation of 9 Gy. Four patients received the conditioning regimen consisting of oral busulfan and intravenous cyclophosphamide. Campath-1G was administered at a daily dose of 5 mg on days -4, -3, -2, -1 and 0. No further GVHD prophylaxis was used. In this study, the overall incidence of grade II-IV acute GVHD was 19%. Graft failure was not observed in this series. Unfortunately, the overall number of patients treated in this study was too small, although further studies appear to be warranted.

A similar attempt for in vivo use of such a monoclonal antibody has been to use anti-CD5 immunotoxin. One such trial, at the University of Minnesota, studied 29 patients with advanced leukemias. The anti-CD5 monoclonal antibody ricin immunotoxin (T101-R) was used for the purpose of GVHD prophylaxis.[70] This monoclonal antibody was used ex vivo. Engraftment was documented in 20 out of 29 patients. At the lower doses of immunotoxin, grade II-IV GVHD occurred in 9 of 10 patients. At the intermediate dose, grade II-IV acute GVHD occurred in 2 of 5 patients and at the highest dose, grade II-IV acute GVHD occurred in 4 of 14 patients. In spite of this in-vitro incubation, the median number of T cells infused was $2.4 \times 10^5$/kg which seems to be higher than the threshold of the T-cell dose associated with the prevention of GVHD. Another immunotoxin, H65 (Xomazyme) has also been used in a large clinical trial. This monoclonal antibody also recognizes the CD5 marker on lymphocytes and is coupled to the ricin A chain. This antibody has been utilized for the prophylaxis of graft-versus-host disease with encouraging results.[71] Another study used Xomazyme in the prophylaxis of GVHD in patients following matched unrelated donor transplantation.[72] This monoclonal antibody has been used with methotrexate and cyclosporine or prednisone. Although this molecule had previously showed potency in prophylaxis of murine GVHD and therapy of human GVHD, in this reported trial the inadequate immunosuppressive potency of these combinations was associated with an unacceptable clinical toxicity. Unfortunately, our experience with this monoclonal antibody for the prophylaxis of acute GVHD in matched unrelated donors has been equally disappointing.

Several other specific T-cell targets have been studied. One promising study is the selective depletion of CD8$^+$ T lymphocytes for the prevention of GVHD. Thirty-six patients undergoing allogeneic bone marrow transplantation from HLA identical siblings had the donor bone marrow treated ex vivo with an anti-CD8 monoclonal antibody and complement.[66] The incidence of grade II-IV acute GVHD was 28% ± 18%. Thirty-three of 36 patients engrafted. The actuarial relapse rate was 11% ± 10% occurring in patients with acute leukemia, but not in patients with chronic myelogenous leukemia. Therefore, this monoclonal antibody appears to retain the graft-versus-leukemia effect as the relapse rate in patients while chronic myelogenous leukemia was not increased. However, the overall incidence of acute GVHD was still high since these patients also received cyclosporine following ex vivo depletion of CD8$^+$ cells. The overall incidence of acute GVHD was not different from that observed in small series using cyclosporine alone.

Another intriguing study performed at the Dana Farber attempted to prevent GVHD by selected depletion of CD6$^+$ T lymphocytes from donor bone marrow.[73] One hundred twelve consecutive adult patients with hematological malignancies undergoing BMT with bone marrow from HLA identical sibling donors were studied. These bone marrows were treated ex vivo with three rounds of incubation with an anti-T12 antibody (anti-CD6) and rabbit complement. Patients received no further prophylactic treatment for acute GVHD. Eighteen percent developed acute GVHD grade II-IV and 2.7% had acute graft failure. These results are encouraging since depletion of CD6$^+$ cells from donor marrow reduced the morbidity and mortality associated with BMT secondary to GVHD. This approach selectively targeted mature T cells but spared closely related and potentially important cells such as NK cells. This may be a reason for the low incidence of graft failure. This particular protocol resulted in a 1.5-2 log depletion of marrow T lymphocytes which could have been sufficient to decrease the occurrence and severity of acute GVHD and at the same time, because of the sparing of NK cells, allowing for early reconstitution.

The low incidence of both graft failure and severe GVHD following transplantation of marrow depleted of T cells by complement-mediated lysis with the antibody against CD6 has been compared to depletion with a mixture of eight antibodies previously used for clinical trials in Seattle.[74]

Possible mechanisms responsible for the difference in the substantial lower risk of graft failure, lymphoid cell surface phenotypes and in vitro function were compared. Treatment with the eight antibody mixture produced a greater than 3 log depletion for precursors of IL-2-producing cells and approximately 1 log depletion of precursors for NK cells. In contrast, treatment with anti-CD6 produced approximately 1 log depletion of precursors for IL-2-producing cells and had no effect on NK precursors. In addition, bone marrow cells remaining after anti-CD6 treatment had more cytotoxic activity when cultured in IL-2 during the first six days of culture. Marrows treated by the two methods showed similar cytotoxicity activity after 10 days in culture. The data lead to the suggestion that a more extensive depletion of T cells and NK cells produced by the eight antibody mixture could result in the higher incidence of graft failure. Thus, it appears that the number of clonogenic T cells present in the graft after T-cell depletion correlates with the development of GVHD.[75]

Another method of T-cell depletion has been by two-step soybean lectin agglutination and sheep red blood cell E-rosette which achieves a 2.5-3 log depletion of clonable T lymphocytes.[76] A study using this technique conducted at Memorial Sloan Kettering enrolled adult patients with acute nonlymphocytic leukemia in first remission receiving related HLA- and MLC-compatible bone marrows. No additional prophylaxis for acute GVHD was used following the T-cell depletion. Thirty-one patients were treated with FTBI and cyclophosphamide for preparation for BMT. Five patients suffered immune-mediated graft rejection and only two patients had grade II acute GVHD. Apparently, these cases of GVHD were limited entirely to skin and resolved promptly, following treatment with steroids. The incidence of acute GVHD was markedly reduced, and clinically apparent chronic GVHD did not occur. All patients had 100% performance status without further immunosuppressive therapy. Unfortunately graft rejection remained a serious limitation to the success of this form of GVHD prophylaxis. Graft failure occurred in 19 of 122 (16%) patients.[77]

Another method of physical manipulation for T-cell depletion is the use of counterflow centrifugal elutriation.[64,78] Two such studies have been reported. In one study, 80 consecutive patients were transplanted with HLA identical sibling marrows for leukemia. The donor marrow was depleted of lymphocytes with counter flow centrifugation. Patients in this trial received methotrexate alone, cyclosporine in combination with methotrexate or cyclosporine alone. Only two patients received no immunoprophylaxis at all. In this study, the probability of acute GVHD $\geq$ grade II was 15%.

However, relapse rates remained problematic, particularly in patients with CML in chronic phase. Overall, the disease-free survival after transplantation for these acute leukemias is not different from data reported at other centers using unmanipulated bone marrow.

In a separate study, 23 patients at Johns Hopkins University received lymphocyte depleted bone marrow allografts, again from HLA identical, MLC nonreactive sibling donors. A standard lymphocyte dose of $5 \times 10^5$ lymphocytes/kg ideal body weight was engineered using the counterflow centrifugal elutriation. Patients were maintained on cyclosporine A immunosuppression for 170 days after BMT. None developed systemic acute GVHD. Moreover, 22 of 23 patients had prompt recovery of hematopoietic cells. Thus, it appears that grafts engineered with counterflow centrifugal elutriation have a low incidence of GVHD and a relatively low incidence of graft failure, but patients must routinely receive additional immunosuppressive agents.

The actual number of T cells is likely to be important. There is a marked decrease in the incidence and severity of acute and chronic GVHD with extensive T-cell depletion of the marrow graft, but a significantly higher incidence of graft failure and relapse of the underlying disease. Investigators in the Netherlands attempted to find an optimal T-cell dose that avoids the extreme risks on both sides.[79] A fixed low number of T cells was utilized. Thirty-one patients received marrow grafts containing $1 \times 10^5$ T cells/kg body weight from HLA identical siblings. All patients received cyclosporine A following transplantation. Engraftment occurred in all patients and no graft rejections were observed. Eight of 30 evaluable patients developed grade II GVHD. One of 13 leukemic transplant recipients relapsed. This suggests that a fixed low number of T cells can allow the graft to "take" and, at the same time, prevent severe GVHD. Unfortunately, the contribution of cyclosporine in this study cannot be ascertained since all but one patient received cyclosporine. A similar trial was performed in children where all bone marrows were T-cell depleted and T-cell addback was prepared for the donor's peripheral blood.[80] The median number of CD3$^+$ cells in this study was $2.6 \times 10^5$/kg recipient weight. These children were not given cyclosporine or methotrexate. There were 14 patients treated, all engrafted, and there were no late graft rejections. Acute GVHD developed in 9 of the 14 children with two children having grade IV GVHD. This study suggests that a high incidence of GVHD can occur in spite of infusion of low numbers of T cells when postgraft immunosuppression is not used. The actual number of T cells to addback in an engineered graft has not been established. It appears from the above study that, at least in children, $2.6 \times 10^5$/kg CD3$^+$ cells are too many. In the adult patient, it appears that one $5 \times 10^5$/kg recipient weight may be safe if cyclosporine is also used.

There has been one prospectively randomized trial in adult leukemic marrow recipients comparing T-cell depletion to cyclosporine and methotrexate, the most commonly utilized drug prophylaxis regimen.[81] Twenty-three patients were randomized to T-cell depletion and 25 patients received cyclosporine and four doses of methotrexate for GVHD prophylaxis. The T-cell depletion method used was an anti-CD8 and an anti-CD6 antibody plus complement. All patients in this trial engrafted except for one patient, who had an early death following transplantation. Patients receiving T cell-depleted marrow had a faster time to engraftment. The incidence of ≥ grade II acute GVHD was 23% following T-cell depletion and 12% for those receiving cyclosporine plus methotrexate. There was no difference in leukemia-free survival. This small study suggests that the drug prophylaxis is as effective as T-cell depletion in the prevention of acute GVHD.

The techniques of monoclonal antibody, in addition to being utilized for prophylaxis of acute GVHD, have been used in the therapy of GVHD. The immunotoxin H65-RTA (Xomazyme) was used in 34 patients who received 14 daily intravenous infusions of immunotoxin for the treatment of acute GVHD.[82] Responses (complete or partial) were seen in 16 of these 34 patients. The highest incidence of response was in patients with skin GVHD, although improvements in the GI tract and liver were also seen. These initial results have been encouraging but these results need to be confirmed by prospective randomized controlled clinical trials (ongoing). A second approach has been to use a murine monoclonal antibody directed against the αβ T-cell receptor in humans.[83] Monoclonal antibody BMA031, which is a murine IgG2b, was used. Seven patients with grade II-III acute GVHD were treated. In five patients a complete and sustained resolution of all disease manifestation was attained while, in one patient, a temporary response was observed. These results, although preliminary, are quite encouraging since such an approach may be useful for the treatment of acute GVHD. Of note, one patient did develop an anti-murine antibody.

Similarly, several studies investigated treatment using an anti-T-cell monoclonal antibody, initially OKT3. The anti-CD3 monoclonal antibody OKT3 is an immunosuppressive, anti-T-cell monoclonal antibody that has been extensively studied in patients. CD3 on T cells is in close contact with the T-cell receptor heterodimer. This complex plays an important role in signal transduction for T cells. Binding of the anti-CD3 monoclonal antibodies induces T-cell receptor signaling in an antigen-independent way. Early studies reported a reduction in GVHD after in vivo treatment of donor marrow with anti-CD3 monoclonal antibody.[60,84] Unfortunately, cases of severe acute GVHD were observed. One difficulty with use of such anti-CD3 is the known cytokine-related morbidity associated with stimulation of these T cells through the CD3 receptor. A study using a rat IgG2 anti-mouse CD3 monoclonal antibody (17A2) suggested that ex vivo treatment of donor cells with 17A2 was not effective.[85] In contrast, conditioning of marrow recipients with a single injection of a 17A2 delayed by one half GVHD mortality by 100 days, and after prolonged treatment, prevented GVHD altogether. These data suggested that purging with anti-T-cell antibodies depends on their Fc part. Moreover, an important anti-CD3 antibody function may be related to its ability to cause downmodulation of the CD3 T-cell receptor complex. In another study, seven patients were treated and two became long-term survivors. OKT3 is accompanied by deterioration of microangiopathy and a prolonged increase of TNF-α serum levels suggesting activation of monocytes and macrophages in vivo.[86] These studies suggest that interference with this or other cytokine release in vivo could potentially improve the clinical responses and decrease the morbidity associated with OKT3. The difficulty with OKT3 is that the treatment was associated with fever, chills, dyspnea, chest pain, wheezing, nausea and vomiting which were more frequent and severe after the first dose.[87,88] OKT3 appears to be an antibody that can mediate cross-linking of the CD3 complex on T cells with Fc receptors and human monocytes. Thus, the Seattle group developed a monoclonal antibody, BC3, which reacts with the CD3 complex but does not interact with the Fc receptors in human monocytes.

An interesting observation has been made of treatment of human or murine lymphocytes with L-leucyl-L-leucine methyl ester (Leu-Leu-OMe).[89] Exposure to this agent results in depletion of all natural killer cells and a fraction of T cells.[90,91] Leu-Leu-OMe is a lysosomotropic peptide that selectively depletes cytotoxic T cells and their precursors, natural killer cells and monocytes, but not helper T cells. Leu-Leu-OMe has been used to deplete cytotoxic T cells and their precursors from human peripheral blood leukocytes and from cells obtained from the peripheral blood, spleen and marrow of other mammalian species used in experimental transplantation studies.[90] Use of this agent in treating the donor marrow and splenocytes in murine models suggests that it is effective in preventing acute GVHD through the first 100 days post-grafting. Similar results were reported in a canine model.[92] Thus, after exposure, B cell and T helper function remains essentially intact whereas the capacity to generate CTLs (CD4$^+$ or CD8$^+$) is abolished. Use of L-leucyl-L-leucine methyl ester results in prevention of lethal GVHD in a parent $\rightarrow$ F$_1$ murine model suggesting that the role of anti-host cytotoxicity is important in this syndrome. However, L-leucyl-L-leucine methyl ester-resistant T cells are fully capable of generating lethal GVHD in a MHC class II disparate strain combination. These findings suggest that a T-cell effector mechanism distinct from the classic cell-mediated cytotoxicity is sufficient to generate lethal GVHD. Incubation of autologous marrow with Leu-Leu-OMe in a canine model had no adverse effects on subsequent engraftment. Incubation of marrow from dog leukocyte antigen of identical litter mates resulted in a higher rate of graft failure. Moreover, incubation of both bone marrow and peripheral blood buffy coats did not prevent the development of GVHD in recipients of marrow from DLA-haplo identical litter mates. These results are clearly less encouraging than those reported using rodent models.

## OTHER METHODS

As mentioned in an earlier section of experimental GVHD, gnotobiosis is an important and effective method to prevent GVHD in murine models. The available data in humans are less clear. For control of infections, protective environment and suppression of gastrointestinal flora have been attempted.[93-95] Part of the problem in comparing different studies is the difficulty in defining what can be considered gnotobiosis in humans. According the data available, gnotobiosis is achieved in mice by removing newborn fetuses into a sterile environment prior to any oral intake and therefore prior to intestinal flora colonization. Once intestinal flora has been established, there is likely to be a continued competition of the various organisms. A major reason for failure is the presence of yeast in surveillance cultures. A second difficulty is to achieve compliance with what can occasionally be a difficult oral regimen. Moreover, there seems to be a delay in the recovery of granulopoiesis in completely decontaminated patients, possibly due to a lower or absent antigenic stimuli with the resultant cytokine release. Some data suggest that complete gnotobiosis in children may help by decreasing morbidity such as severe infections and GVHD.[96]

Another method attempted to prevent GVHD, that follows the reasoning of gnotobiosis, is to decrease gram-negative bacteria using antibodies. One hypothesis for the efficacy of gnotobiosis is that bacterial endotoxin can activate monocytes and macrophages to release IL-1, TNF and γ-interferon, all of which can lead to or enhance T-cell proliferation. Endotoxin is a lipopolysaccharide that may enter the blood stream, especially if the GI tract is denuded from the high dose therapy prior to transplantation or from methotrexate used in the prophylaxis of GVHD. An attempt to modulate these gram-negative organisms was performed by using an immunoglobulin enriched for IgM (Pentaglobulin). Pentaglobulin contains antibodies that are active against these organisms.[97] The results suggest that this particular antibody formulation may have some effect on mild to moderate GVHD.

## NEWER AGENTS

The unique difference in allogeneic bone marrow transplantation compared to organ transplantation is that immunosuppression is needed in both directions. That is, the host must be suppressed so that the graft is not rejected, but at the same time, the graft must also be suppressed so as not to cause GVHD. Newer selective immunosuppressents are on the horizon. One pathway for immunosuppression is to specifically affect activated lymphocytes, especially T cells. Since antigen-activated T (and B) cells depend on purine de novo synthesis, whereas most other cells can utilize the salvage pathway, inhibition of purine synthesis may be an attractive approach. A study to evaluate the possibility of using 2-deoxy-chloro adenosine (2-CdA) for the prophylaxis and treatment of GVHD would be interesting.

Another new immunosuppressant appears to be mycophenolate mofetil, also known as RS-61443, an ester product of mycophenolic acid that inhibits de novo synthesis of guanine nucleotides.[98] This drug apparently was useful in preventing GVHD after allogeneic rat small bowel transplants. More importantly, it gave the recipient long-term tolerance against GVHD after discontinuation of therapy.[99]

Trimetrexate is a 2,4-diaminoquinazoline folate analog synthesized in the early 1970s as an anti-malarial agent.[100] Similar to methotrexate, trimetrexate is a potent inhibitor of the enzyme dihydrofolate reductase. Unlike methotrexate, trimetrexate is not excreted in the urine, but rather is metabolized by the liver. Because of this, a trial was conducted in dogs to investigate whether trimetrexate would be superior to methotrexate.[101] The rationale for this was cyclosporines' known nephrotoxicity and that disposal of methotrexate relies predominantly on renal excretion. Ten dogs received total body irradiation followed by marrow and buffy coat cells from litter mate donors differing by one DLA haplotype. The results achieved with trimetrexate and cyclosporine is roughly equivalent to the results achieved with the combination of methotrexate and cyclosporine in similar mismatched donor recipient pairs. This suggests the substitution of methotrexate by trimetrexate can be made. In an initial phase I study in humans, trimetrexate was well-tolerated at doses of 120-200 mg/m$^2$ as a single dose.[100]

FK506 has been found to be as effective as cyclosporine for the prevention of rejection of cell or organ allografts and is potentially less toxic.[102] FK506 has been used extensively in animal models. In a comparison study between FK506 and cyclosporine, FK506 appeared to be more effective but there was delayed appearance of GVHD after discontinuation of treatment.[103] However, small doses of maintenance FK506 every other day suppressed GVHD once the induction period was completed. FK506 can also reverse established GVHD in an experimental model[104] as well as ameliorate chronic GVHD in humans.[105]

A second approach using FK506 is donor pre-treatment with FK506. This appears to prevent acute GVHD after allogeneic BMT.[106] A study using FK506 for donor treatment only, as well as in combination with recipient treatment, was performed. A single dose of FK506 given to the allogeneic bone marrow donor can significantly prolong the mean GVHD-free interval after allogeneic BMT. The results were clearly better when combined with recipient course of FK506. Explanations for efficacy of donor pretreatment may be related to drug carryover versus a direct effect on the donor cells prior to BMT.

Deoxyspergualin is a new immunosuppressive agent. It is a derivative of spergualin and is isolated from culture filtrates of bacillus laterosporus.[107] Deoxyspergualin abolishes the activity of cytotoxic T lymphocytes, not only at the induction stage, but also at the advanced stages of the disease. Deoxyspergualin can inhibit alloreactive cytotoxic activity in GVHD.[108] Deoxyspergualin can also decrease the development of lethal GVHD and the generation of alloreactive cytotoxic activity. Various experiments[109] demonstrate that bone marrow and spleen cells from deoxyspergualin-treated survivors lacked the ability to induce lethal GVHD. These results suggest that the survivors have immunological unresponsiveness. The findings also suggest that suppressor cells with the ability to suppress development of GVHD are present in the lymph node cells of survivors. These cells may play an important role in maintenance of immunological unresponsiveness. Deoxyspergualin has also been combined with methotrexate and appears to be even more effective than using either alone.[110]

Ex vivo use of spermine dialdehyde treatment in a murine bone marrow transplantation model is another method to prevent lethal GVHD. Spermine dialdehyde is an oxidized product of spermine, which is identified to be an immunosuppressive factor. Spermine dialdehyde was found to be a potent irreversible suppressor of T-cell functions. Studies indicate that pre-treatment of bone marrow grafts with spermine dialdehyde modulated GVHD after allogeneic BMT in a murine model.[111] Data demonstrate that ex vivo treatment of histoincompatible bone marrow grafts with spermine dialdehyde effectively prevents GVHD in a lethally irradiated mouse model. In vitro assays demonstrated that spermine dialdehyde can inactivate T cells and NK cells or spermine myeloid cells which are required for reconstitution.

Another new immunosuppressive agent is rapamycin. Rapamycin is a related macrolide to FK-506. These related macrolides act as reciprocal antagonists in T cells.[112,113] Rapamycin has been used to suppress both host-versus-graft and graft-versus-host disease in MHC-mismatched rats.[114] The use of rapamycin resulted in significant suppression in both host-versus-graft and graft-versus-host reaction after small bowel transplantation in rats.

Studies in a murine model show UVB irradiation of lymphoid hematopoietic cells results in the prevention of GVHD.[115] Use of UVB light appears to selectively inhibit lymphocyte function while preserving hematopoietic colony formation. UVB irradiation of spleen cells added to normal marrow cells prevented the development of GVHD. A number of mice became complete donor-type chimeras. Mice without GVHD showed specific tolerance of skin grafts from a second parent strain, while animals with GVHD rejected the skin grafts. UVB may induce tolerance through elimination of a co-stimulatory factor. UVB modifies class II antigen expression of the cell surface and can also help alter calcium homeostasis.[116,117] Moreover, UVB exposure may result in activation of apoptosis leading to specific cell death of activated cell populations.

More data suggest that sensitization of UV-irradiated mice with allogeneic cells does induce specific suppression of allograft rejection.[118] The induction of GVHD is also suppressed by this treatment. Suppressor T cells can be found in the spleen of UV-irradiated, antigen-sensitized mice. This suggests that antigen-specific suppressor T cells present in the spleens of UV irradiated alloantigen-sensitized mice suppress the immune response against such alloantigens.

Cell surface glycoproteins are known to play an important part in lymphocyte interactions. Therefore modification of these structures to impair lymphocyte interactions and therefore interfere with the development of GVHD have been attempted. Neuraminidase pretreatment of donor lymphocytes decreased the incidence of acute GVHD.[119] Treatment with neuraminidase did not compromise engraftment and had no adverse effect on T-cell or B-cell function following adoptive transfer experiments. Although the exact mechanism by which this treatment prevents GVHD is unknown, the data suggest it does provide such protection.

Another potential agent is gliotoxin.[120] Gliotoxin is a member of the epipolythiodioxopiperazine family of secondary fungal metabolites. Gliotoxin inhibits a variety of biological functions of cells of the reticulo-endothelial system. In particular, gliotoxin is able to inhibit mitogen- and interleukin-mediated proliferation and interleukin released by mature lymphocytes. Treatment of allogeneic spleen cells with gliotoxin allows the transfer into sublethally irradiated recipients without inducing a graft-versus-host reaction. Gliotoxin treatment resulted in the establishment of fully allogeneic bone marrow chimeras free of GVHD. However, immune competence is severely compromised in these mice by the lack of donor MHC-type stimulator cells.

Other potential immunosuppressive agents under development include SK&K 105685, a novel azaspirane that has an immunomodulatory and therapeutic activity in animal models without immune disease.[121] This agent appears to induce nonspecific suppressor cell activity in vivo and is able to prolong vascularized cardiac allograft survival in rats. This agent has not been tried in GVHD.

## REFERENCES

1. Sullivan K, Deeg HJ, Sanders A et al. Hyperacute graft-versus-host disease in patients not given immunosuppression after allogeneic marrow transplantation. Blood 1986; 67: 1172.

2. Lazarus H, Coccia PF, Herzig RH et al. Incidence of acute graft-versus-host disease with and without methotrexate prophylaxis in allogeneic bone marrow transplantation. Blood 1984; 64: 215.

3. Elfenbein G, Goedect T, Graham-Pole J, Skoda-Smith S, Gross S, Weiner R. Is prophylaxis against acute graft-versus-host disease necessary if treatment is effective and survival is not empaired? Proc Am Soc Clin Oncol 1986; 5: 643.

4. Uphoff D. Alteration of homograft reaction by α-methopterin in lethally irradiated mice treated with homologous marrow. Proc Soc Exp Biol Med 1958; 99: 651.

5. Storb R, Epstein RB, Graham TC, Thomas ED. Methotrexate regimens for control of graft-versus-host disease in dogs with allogeneic marrow grafts. Transplantation 1970; 9: 240.

6. Santos G, Owens AH. Production of graft-versus-host disease in the rat and its treatment with cytotoxic agents. Nature 1966; 210: 139.

7. Storb R, Deeg HJ, Fisher L et al. Cyclosporine v methotrexate for graft-v-host disease prevention in patients given marrow grafts for leukemia: Long-term follow-up of three controlled trials. Blood 1988; 71: 293.

8. Santos G, Tutschka PJ, Brookmeyer R et al. Cyclosporine plus methylprednisolone versus cyclophosphamide plus methylprednisolone as prophylaxis for graft-versus-host disease: A randomized double-blind study in patients undergoing allogeneic marrow transplantation. Clin Transplantation 1987; 1: 21.

9. Weiden P, Doney K, Storb R, Thomas ED. Anti-human thymocyte globulin prophylaxis of acute graft-versus-host disease: A randomized trial in patients with leukemia treated with HLA-identical sibling matched grafts. Transplantation 1979; 27: 227.

10. Doney K, Weiden PL, Storb R, Thomas ED. Failure of early administration of antithymocyte globulin to lessen graft-versus-host disease in human allogeneic marrow transplant recipients. Transplantation 1981; 31: 141.

11. Ramsay N, Kersey J, Robison LL et al. A randomized study of the prevention of acute graft-versus-host disease. N Engl J Med 1982; 306: 392.

12. Tutschka P, Beschorner WE, Allison AC, Burns WH, Santos GW. Use of cyclosporin A in allogeneic bone marrow transplantation in rats. Nature 1979; 280: 148.

13. Tutschka P, Beschorner WE, Hess AD, Santos GW. Cyclosporine A to prevent graft-versus-host disease: A pilot study in 22 patients receiving allogeneic marrow transplant. Blood 1983; 61: 318.

14. Powles R, Clink HM, Spence D et al. Cyclosporin A to prevent graft-versus-host disease in man after allogeneic bone marrow transplantation. Lancet 1980; 1: 327.

15. Deeg H, Storb R, Thomas ED et al. Cyclosporine as prophylaxis for graft-versus-host disease: A randomized study in patients undergoing marrow transplantation for acute nonlymphoblastic leukemia. Blood 1985; 65: 1325.

16. Santos G, Brookmeyer R, Saral R, Tutschka PJ. Cyclosporine (CsA) versus cyclophosphamide (CY): Prevention of graft-versus-host disease (GVHD). Exp Hematol 1985; 13: 427.

17. Storb R, Deeg HJ, Pepe M et al. Long-term follow-up of three controlled trials comparing cyclosporine versus methotrexate for graft-verus-host disease prevention in patients given marrow grafts for leukemia. Blood 1992; 79: 3091.

18. Backman L, Ringden O, Tollemar J, Lonnqvist B. An increased risk of relapse in cyclosporin-treated compared with methotrexate-treated patients: Long-term follow-up of a randomized trial. Bone Marrow Transpl 1988; 3: 463.

19. Ruutu T, Volin L, Elonen E. Low incidence of severe acute and chronic graft-versus-host disease as a result of prolonged cyclosporine prophylaxis and early aggressive treatment with corticosteroids. Transpl Proc 1988; 20: 491.

20. Deeg HJ, Storb R, Appelbaum FR, Kennedy MS, Graham TC, Thomas ED. Combined immunosuppression with cyclosporine and methotrexate in dogs given bone marrow grafts from DLA haploidentical littermates. Transplantation 1984; 37: 62.

21. Deeg H, Storb R, Weiden PL et al. Cyclosporin A and methotrexate in canine marrow transplantation: Engraftment, graft-versus-host disease, and induction of tolerance. Transplantation 1982; 34: 30.

22. Ringden O, Klaesson S, Sundberg B, Ljungman P, Lonnqvist B, Persson U. Decreased incidence of graft-versus-host disease and improved survival with methotrexate combined with cyclosporin compared with monotherapy in recipients of bone marrow from donors other that HLA identical siblings. Bone Marrow Transpl 1992; 9: 19.

23. Mrsic M, Labar B, Boganic V et al. Combination of cyclosporin and methotrexate for prophylaxis of acute graft-versus-host disease after allogeneic bone marrow transplantation for leukemia. Bone Marrow Transpl 1990; 6: 137.

24. Gluckman E, Horowitz MM, Champlin RE et al. Bone marrow transplantation for severe aplastic anemia: Influence of conditioning and graft-versus-host disease prophylaxis regimens on outcome. Blood 1992; 79: 269.

25. Storb R, Deeg HJ, Farewell V et al. Marrow transplantation for severe aplastic anemia: Methotrexate alone compared with a combination of methotrexate and cyclosporine for prevention of acute graft-versus-host disease. Blood 1986; 68: 119.

26. Storb R, Deeg HJ, Whitehead J et al. Methotrexate and cyclosporine compared with cyclosporine alone for prophylaxis of acute graft-versus-host disease after marrow transplantation for leukemia. N Engl J Med 1986; 314: 729.

27. Storb R, Deeg HJ, Whitehead J et al. Marrow transplantation for leukemia and aplastic anemia: Two controlled trials of a combination of methotrexate and cyclosporine v cyclosporine alone or methotrexate alone for prophylaxis of acute graft-v-host disease. Transpl Proc 1987; 19: 2608.

28. Storb R, Deeg HJ, Pepe M et al. Methotrexate and cyclosporine versus cyclosporine alone for prophylaxis of graft-versus-host disease in patients given HLA-identical marrow grafts for leukemia: Long-term follow-up of a controlled trial. Blood 1989; 73: 1729.

29. Marks D, Hughes TP, Szydlo R et al. HLA-identical sibling donor bone marrow transplantation for chronic myeloid leukemia in first chronic phase: influence of GVHD prophylaxis on outcome. Br J Haematol 1992; 81: 383.

30. Beelen D, Quabeck K, Kaiser B et al. Six weeks of continuous intravenous cyclosporine and short-course methotrexate as prophylaxis for acute graft-versus-host disease after allogeneic bone marrow transplantation. Transplantation 1990; 50: 421.

31. Stockschlaeder M, Storb R, Pepe M et al. A pilot study of low-dose cyclosporin for graft-versus-host prophylaxis in marrow transplantation. Br J Haematol 1992; 80: 49.

32. Forman S, Blume KG, Krance RA et al. A prospective randomized study of acute graft-vs-host disease in 107 patients with leukemia: methotrexate/prednisone vs cyclosporin a/prednisone. Transplant Proc 1987; 19: 2605.

33. Chao NJ, Schmidt GM, Niland JC et al. Cyclosporine, methotrexate, and prednisone compared with cyclosporine and prednisone for prophylaxis of acute graft-versus-host disease. N. Engl J Med 1993; 329:1225.

34. Martin P, Schoch G, Fisher L et al. A retrospective analysis of therapy for acute graft-versus-host disease: Secondary treatment. Blood 1991; 77: 1821.

35. Tutschka P, Copelan EA, Klein JP. Bone marrow transplantation for leukemia following a new busulfan and cyclophosphamide regimen. Blood 1987; 70: 1382.

36. Yau J, LeMaistre CF, Zagars GK et al. Methylprednisone, cyclosporine and methotrexate for prophylaxis for acute graft-versus-host disease. Bone Marrow Transpl 1990; 5: 269.

37. Biggs J, Szer J, Crilley P et al. Treatment of chronic myeloid leukemia with allogeneic bone marrow transplantation after preparation with BuCy2. Blood 1992; 80: 1352.

38. Blume K, Kopecky K, Henslee-Doney J et al. A prospective randomized comparison of total body irradiation-etoposide versus busulfan-cyclophosphamide as preparatory regimens for bone marrow transplantation in patients who were not in first remission: A Southwest Oncology Group Study. Blood 1993; 81: 2187.

39. Storb R, Pepe M, Anasetti C et al. What role for prednisone in prevention of acute graft-versus-host disease in patients undergoing marrow transplants? Blood 1990; 76: 1037.

40. Schmidt G, Niland JC, Forman SJ et al. Extended follow-up in 212 long-term allogeneic bone marrow transplant survivors: Addressing issues of quality of life. Transplantation 1992; 55: 551.

41. Atkinson K, Biggs J, Concannon A et al. A prospective randomised trial of cyclosporin and methotrexate versus cyclosporin, methotrexate and prednisolone for prevention of graft-versus-host disease after HLA-identical sibling marrow transplantation for haematological malignancy. Aust NZ J Med 1991; 21: 850.

42. Nash R, Pepe MS, Storb R et al. Acute graft-versus-host disease: Analysis of risk factors after allogeneic marrow transplantation and prophylaxis with cyclosporine and methotrexate. Blood 1992; 80: 1838.

43. Tollemar J, Ringden O, Backman L et al. Results of four different protocols for prophylaxis against graft-versus-host disease. Transpl Proc 1989; 21: 3008.

44. Essell J, Thompson JM, Harman GS. Marked increase in veno-occlusive disease of the liver associated with methotrexate use for graft-versus-host disease prophylaxis in patients receiving busulfan/cyclophosphamide. Blood 1992; 79: 2784.

45. Atkinson K, Downs K, Ashby M, Biggs J. Clinical correlations with cyclosporine blood levels after allogeneic bone marrow transplantation: An analysis of four different assays. Transpl Proc 1990; 22: 1331.

46. Hunter A, Besell EM, Rusell NH. Effective prevention of acute GVHD following allogeneic BMT with low leukemic relapse using methotrexate and therapeutically monitored levels of cyclosporin A. Bone Marrow Transplant 1992; 10: 431.

47. Deeg HJ, Loughran TP Jr, Storb R et al. Treatment of human acute graft-

versus-host disease with anti-thymocyte globulin and cyclosporine with or without methylprednisolone. Transplantation 1985; 401: 1626.

48. Smith K. The interleukin-2 receptor. In: Advances in Immunology. Vol 42. New York: Academic Press, 1988: 165.

49. Anasetti C, Martin PJ, Storb R et al. Prophylaxis of graft-versus-host disease by administration of the murine anti-IL-2 receptor antibody 2A3. Bone Marrow Transpl 1991; 7: 375.

50. Blaise D, Olive D, Hirn M et al. Prevention of acute GVHD by in vivo use of anti-interleukin-2 receptor monoclonal antibody (33B3.1): A feasibility trial in 15 patients. Bone Marrow Transpl 1991; 8: 105.

51. Davignon D, Martz E, Reynolds T et al. Monoclonal antibody to a novel lymphocyte function-associated (LFA-1): Mechanisms of blockade of T lymphocyte-mediated killing and effects on other T and B lymphocyte functions. J Immunol 1981; 127: 590.

52. Krensky A, Sanchez-Madrid F, Robbins E et al. The functional significance, distribution, and structure of LFA-1; LFA-2; and LFA-3: Cell surface antigens associated with CTL-target interactions. J Immunol 1983; 131: 611.

53. Harning R, Pelletier J, Lubbe K, Takei F, Merluzzi VJ. Reduction in the severity of graft-versus-host disease and increased survival in allogeneic mice by treatment with monoclonal antibodies to cell adhesion antigens LFA-1α and MALA-2. Transplantation 1991; 52: 842.

54. Schlegel P, Vaysburg M, Chao NJ. Selective inhibition of T-cell costimulation mediated by VCAM-1 prevents murine graft-versus-host disease. Blood 1993; 82: 456a.

55. Sheridan J, Tutschka PJ, Sedmak DD et al. Immunoglobulin G subclass deficiency and pneumococcal infection after allogeneic bone marrow transplantation. Blood 1990; 75: 1583.

56. Aucouturier P, Barra A, Intrator L et al. Long-lasting IgG subclass and antibacterial polysaccharide antibody deficiency after allogeneic bone marrow transplantation. Blood 1987; 70: 779.

57. Sullivan K, Kopecky KJ, Jocom J et al. Immunomodulatory and antimicrobial efficacy of intravenous immunoglobulin in bone marrow transplantation. N Engl J Med 1990; 323: 705.

58. Prentice H, Janossy G, Trejdosiewicz L et al. Depletion of T lymphocytes in donor marrow prevents significant graft-versus-host disease in matched allogeneic leukemic marrow transplant recipients. Lancet 1984; 1: 472.

59. Mitsuyasu R, Champlin RE, Gale RP et al. Treatment of donor bone marrow with monoclonal anti-T-cell antibody and complement for the prevention of graft-versus-host disease. Ann Intern Med 1986; 105: 20.

60. Fillipovich A, McGlave PB, Ramsay NKC et al. Pretreatment of donor bone marrow with monoclonal antibody OKT3 for prevention of acute graft-versus-host disease in allogeneic histocompatible bone marrow transplantation. Lancet 1982; 1: 1266.

61. Antin J, Bierer B, Smith BR et al. Selective depletion of bone marrow T lymphocytes with anti-CD5 monoclonal antibodies: Effective prophylaxis for graft-versus-host disease in patients with hematologic malignancies. Blood 1991; 78: 2139.

62. Hale G, Cobbold SP, Waldman H. For Campath-1 Users, T-cell depletion with Campath-1 in allogeneic bone marrow transplantation. Transplantation 1988; 45: 753.

63. Reisner Y, O'Reilly RJ, Kapoor N et al. Allogeneic bone marrow transplantation using stem cells fractionated by lectins: In vitro analysis of soybean agglutinin. Lancet 1980; 2: 1320.

64. Wagner J, Santos GW, Noga SJ et al. Bone marrow graft engineering by counterflow centrifugal elutriation: Results of a phase I-II clinical trial. Blood 1990; 75: 1370.

65. Goldman J, Gale RP, Bortin MM et al. Bone marrow transplantation for chronic myelogenous leukemia in chronic phase: Increased risk of relapse associated with T-cell depletion. Ann Intern Med 1988; 108: 806.

66. Champlin R, Ho W, Gajewski J et al. Selective depletion of CD8+ T lymphocytes for prevention of graft-versus-host disease after allogeneic bone marrow transplantation. Blood 1990; 76: 418.

67. Martin P, Hansen JA, Buckner CD et al. Effects of in vitro depletion of T cells in HLA-identical allogeneic marrow grafts. Blood 1985; 66: 664.

68. Maraninchi D, Blaise D, Rio B et al. Impact of T-cell depletion on outcome of allogeneic bone-marrow transplantation for standard-risk leukemias. Lancet 1987; 2: 175.

69. Willemze R, Richel DJ, Falkenburg JHF et al. In vivo use of Campath-1G to prevent graft-versus-host disease and graft rejection after bone marrow transplantation. Bone Marrow Transpl 1992; 9: 255.

70. Fillipovich A, Vallera D, McGlave P et al. T-cell depletion with anti-CD5 immunotoxin in histocompatible bone marrow transplantatin. Transplantation 1990; 50: 410.

71. Henslee-Downey P, Pettigrew AL, Schmitt F et al. The use of alternative donors for marrow transplantation in the correction of Hurler's syndrome. Blood 1990; 76: 544a.

72. Weisdorf D, Filipovich A, McGlave P et al. Combination graft-versus-host disease prophylaxis using immunotoxin (anti-CD5-RTA [Xomazyme-CD5]) plus methotrexate and cyclosporine or prednisone after unrelated donor marrow transplantation. Bone Marrow Transplant 1993; 12: 531.

73. Soiffer R, Murray C, Mauch P et al. Prevention of graft-versus-host disease by selective depletion of CD6 positive T lymphocytes from donor bone marrow. J Clin Oncol 1992; 10: 1191.

74. Voltarelli J, Corpuz S, Martin PJ. In vitro comparison of two methods of T-cell depletion associated with different rates of graft failure after allogeneic marrow transplantation. Bone Marrow Transpl 1990; 6: 419.

75. Kernan N, Collins NH, Juliano L, Cartagena T, Dupont B, O'Reilly RJ. Clonable T lymphocytes in T-cell depleted bone marrow transplants correlate with development of graft-versus-host disease. Blood 1986; 68: 770.

76. Young J, Papadopoulos EB, Cunningham I et al. T-cell depleted allogeneic bone marrow transplantation in adults with acute nonlymphocyctic leukemia in first remission. Blood 1992; 79: 3380.

77. Kernan N, Bordignon C, Heller G et al. Graft failure after T-cell-depleted human leukocyte antigen identical marrow transplants for leukemia: I. Analysis of risk factors and results of secondary transplants. Blood 1989; 74: 2227.

78. Schattenberg A, De Witte T, Preijers F et al. Allogeneic bone marrow transplantation for leukemia with marrow grafts depleted of lymphocytes by counterflow centrifugation. Blood 1990; 75: 1356.

79. Verdonck L, de Gast GC, van Heugten HG, Dekker AW. A fixed low number of T cells in HLA-identical allogeneic bone marrow transplantation.

Blood 1990; 75: 776.

80. Potter M, Pamphilon DH, Cornish JM, Oakhill A. Graft-versus-host disease in children receiving HLA-identical allogeneic bone marrow transplants with a low adjusted T lymphocyte dose. Bone Marrow Transpl 1991; 8: 357

81. Ringden O, Pihlstedt P, Marking L et al. Prevention of graft-versus-host disease with T-cell depletion or cyclosporin and methotrexate: A randomized trial in adult leukemic marrow recipients. Bone Marrow Transpl 1991; 7: 221.

82. Byers V, Henslee PJ, Kernan NA et al. Use of anti-pan T-lymphocyte ricin A chain immunotoxin in steroid-resistant acute graft-versus-host disease. Blood 1990; 75:1426.

83. Beelen D, Grosse-Wilde H, Ryscha U et al. Initial treatment of acute graft-versus-host disease with a murine monoclonal antibody directed to the human α/β T-cell receptor. Cancer Immunol Immunolther 1991; 34: 97.

84. Prentice H, Blacklock HA, Janossy G et al. Use of anti-T-cell monoclonal antibody OKT3 to prevent acute graft-versus-host disease in allogeneic bone-marrow transplantation for acute leukaemia. Lancet 1982; 1: 700.

85. Mysliwietz J, Thierfelder S. Antilymphocytic antibodies and marrow transplantation. XII: Suppresion of graft-versus-host disease by T-cell-modulating and depleting antimouse CD3 antibody is most effective when preinjected in the marrow recipient. Blood 1992; 80: 2661.

86. Gleixner B, Kolb HJ, Holler E et al. Treatment of a GVHD with OKT3: Clinical outcome and side-effects associated with release of TNFα. Bone Marrow Transpl 1991; 8: 93.

87. Martin P, Hansen JA, Anasetti C et al. Treatment of acute graft-versus-host disease with anti-CD3 monoclonal antibodies. Am J Kidney Dis 1988; 11: 149.

88. Gratama J, Jansen J, Lipovich RA, Tanke HJ, Goldstein G, Zwaan FE. Treatment of acute graft-versus-host disease with anti-CD3 monoclonal antibodies. AM J Kidney Dis 1988; 11: 152.

89. Thiele D, Bryde SE, Lipsky PE. Lethal graft-versus-host-disease induced by a class II MHC antigen only disparity is not mediated by cytotoxic T cells. J Immunol 1988; 141: 3377.

90. Thiele D, Lipsky, PE. The immunosuppressive activity of L-leucyl-L-leucine methyl ester: selective ablation of cytotoxic lymphocytes and monocytes. J Immunol 1986; 136: 1038.

91. Thiele D, Charley MR, Calomeni JA, Lipsky PE. Lethal graft-vs-host disease across major histocompatibility barriers: requirement for leucyl-leucine methyl ester sensitive cytotoxic T cells. J Immunol 1987; 138: 51.

92. Raff R, Severns EM, Storb R et al. Studies on the use of L-leucyl-L-leucine methyl ester in canine allogeneic marrow transplantation. Transplantation 1992; 55: 1244.

93. Buckner C, Clift RA, Sanders JE et al. Protective enviroment for marrow transplant recipients. A prospective study. Ann Int Med 1978; 89: 893.

94. Levine A, Siegel SE, Schreiber AD et al. Protected enviroments and prophylactic antibiotics. A prospective controlled study on their utility in the therapy of acute leukemia. N Engl J Med 1973; 288: 477.

95. Schimpff S, Greene WH, Young VM et al. Infection prevention in acute nonlymphoblastic leukemia. Laminar air flow reverse isolation with oral, nonabsorbable antibiotic prophylaxis. Ann Int Med 1975; 82: 351.

96. Vossen J, Heidt PJ, van den Berg H, Gerritsen EJA, Hermans J, Dooren LJ. Prevention of infection and graft-versus-host disease by suppression of intestinal microflora in children treated with allogeneic bone marrow transplantation. Eur J Clin Micro Inf 1990; 9: 14.

97. Klingemann H, Barnett MJ, Reece DE, Shepherd JD, Phillips GL. Use of an immunoglobulin preparation enriched for IgM (pentaglobin)for the treatment of acute graft-versus-host disease. Bone Marrow Transpl 1990; 6: 199.

98. Allison A, Almquist SJ, Muller CD, Eugui EM. In vitro immunosuppressive effects of mycophenolic acid and an ester pro-drug RS-61443. Transplant Proc 1991; 23: 10.

99. Sonnino R. RS-61443 prevents graft-versus-host disease but not rejection in allogeneic rat small bowel transplants. Transpl Proc 1992; 24: 1190.

100. Lin J, Bertino JR. Trimetrexate: a second generation folate antagonist in clinical trial. J Clin Oncol 1987; 5: 2032.

101. Appelbaum F, Raff RF, Storb R et al. Use of trimetrexate for the prevention of graft-versus-host disease. Bone Marrow Transpl 1989; 4: 421.

102. Thomson A. FK-506 enters the clinic. Immunol Today 1990; 11: 35.

103. Markus P, Cai X, Ming W, Demetris AJ, Fung JJ, Starzl TE. Prevention of graft-versus-host disease following allogeneic bone marrow transplantation in rate using FK506. Transplantation 1991; 52: 590.

104. Markus P, Cai X, Ming W, Demetris AJ, Fung JJ, Starzl TE. FK 506 reverses acute graft-versus-host disease following allogeneic bone marrow transplantation in rats. Surgery 1991; 110: 357.

105. Fung J, Todo S, Tzakis AG et al. Current status of FK 506 in liver transplantation. Transplant Proc 1991; 23: 1902.

106. Cooper M, Markus PM, Cai X, Starzl TE, Fung JJ. Prolonged prevention of acute graft-versus-host disease after allogeneic bone marrow transplantation by donor pretreatment using FK 506. Transpl Proc 1991; 23: 3238.

107. Takeuchi T, Iinuma H, Kunimoto S et al. A new anti-tumor antibiotic spergualin: isolation and antitumor activity. J Antibiot 1981; 34: 1619.

108. Nemoto K, Hayashi M, Abe F, Takita T, Takeuchi T. Inhibition by deoxyspergualin of allo-reactive cytotoxic activity in M graft-versus-host disease. Transpl Proc 1989; 21: 3028.

109. Nemoto K, Sugawara Y, Mae T et al. Immunological unresponsiveness by deoxyspergualin therapy in mice undergoing lethal graft-vs-host disease, and successful adoptive transfer of unresponsiveness. Transpl Proc 1991; 23: 862.

110. Nemoto K, Hayshi M, Ito J et al. Deoxyspergualin in lethal murine graft-versus-host disease. Transplantation 1991; 51: 712.

111. Wang E, Mason Conant J, Li D, Viscounti V, Chourmouzis E, Lau C. Ex vivo spermine dialdehyde treatment prevents lethal GVHD in a murine bone marrow transplantation model. Bone Marrow Transpl 1990; 6: 235.

112. Dumont F, Melino MR, Staruch MJ et al. The immunosuppressive macrolides FK-506 and rapamycin act as reciprocal antagonists in murine T cells. J Immunol 1990; 144: 1418.

113. Dumont F, Staruch MJ, Koprak SL et al. Distinct mechanisms of suppression of murine T-cell activation by the related macrolides FK-506 and rapamycin. J Immunol 1990; 144: 251.

114. Fabian M, Denning SM, Bollinger RR. Rapamycin suppression of host-versus-graft and graft-versus-host disease in MHC-mismatched rats. Transplant Proc 1992; 24: 1174.

115. Cohn M, Cahill RA, Deep HJ. Hematopoietic reconstitution and prevention of graft-versus-host disease with UVB-irradiated haploidentical murine spleen and marrow cells. Blood 1991; 78: 3317.

116. Deeg HJ, Sigaroudinia M. Ultraviolet B-induced loss of HLA class II antigen expression on lymphocytes is dose, time, and locus dependent. Exp Hematol 1990; 18: 916.

117. Spielberg H, June CH, Blair OC, Nystrim-Rosander C, Cereb N, Deeg HJ. Ultraviolet-irradiation of lymphocytes triggers increase in intracellular $CA^{2+}$ and prevents lectin-stimulated $CA^{2+}$ mobilization: Evidence for UV and nifedipine sensitive calcium channels. Exp Hematol 1991 19: 742.

118. Ullrich S, Magee, M. Specific suppression of allograft rejection after treatment of recipient mice with ultraviolet radiation and allogeneic spleen cells. Transplantation 1988; 46: 115.

119. Stacey N, Cox J, Loblay R, Crosbie J. Neuraminidase pretreatment of donor lymphocytes and graft-versus-host disease. Int Soc Exp Hemat 1989; 17: 273.

120. Mullbacher A, Moreland AF, Waring P, Sjaarda, A, Eichner, RD. Prevention of graft-versus-host disease by treatment of bone marrow with gliotoxin in fully allogeneic chimeras and their cytotoxic T-cell repertoire. Transplantation 1988; 46: 120.

121. Schmidbauer G, Hancock WW, Badger AM, Kupiec-Weglinski JW. Induction of nonspecific X-irradiation-resistant suppressor cell activity in vivo and prolongation of vascularized allograft survival by SK&F 105685: A novel immunomodulatory azaspirane. Transplantation 1993; 55: 1236.

# TREATMENT OF ACUTE GVHD

## STEROIDS

The first line of therapy following failure of GVHD prophylaxis is the use of glucocorticoids (steroids). The mechanism of action of the glucocorticoids is presumably related to the lympholytic effects. In fact, all therapies attempted for treatment of acute GVHD had been administered only for "steroid-resistant" disease. High dose steroids have been used, for example, as high as 20 mg/kg/day for three days with a taper, with occasional prompt responses. However, recrudescence was observed with dose reduction.[1] Another regimen using high-dose methylprednisolone up to 500 mg/m$^2$ every six hours was also attempted. Despite responses, all of the long-term survivors developed chronic GVHD.[2] Most of the failures from these regimens have been secondary to opportunistic infection or interstitial pneumonitis. A more moderate dose increase to 1.5-2 mg/kg has also been used.[3] Patients with mild to moderate GVHD had an excellent response, while patients with severe GVHD did poorly. Successful therapy of acute GVHD did not affect the risk of leukemic relapse.[4]

A group in Minnesota analyzed the long-term outcome of patients who were treated for grade II-IV acute GVHD following histocompatible allogeneic BMT.[5] Out of 469 patients receiving allogeneic BMT, 179 (42%) developed grade II or greater acute GVHD. Seventy-two patients (41%) achieved complete or continued resolution of acute GVHD after a median of 21 days of therapy. Treatment for these responders consisted primarily of corticosteroids or other immunosuppressive therapies including cyclosporine A, anti-T-cell immunotoxin or anti-lymphocyte globulin. Patients not responding to these initial immunosuppressive agents received high-dose methylprednisolone, anti-thymocyte globulin with steroids or other therapies because of refractory or progressive symptoms of acute GVHD. Only 7of these 61 patients eventually attained a complete continued remission. The overall rate of chronic GVHD in this group who had suffered acute GVHD was 70%. More favorable responses to therapy occurred in patients without liver or skin involvement, patients with acute lymphoblastic leukemia and donor/recipient pairs other than male patients with female donors. Although these results are quite good, suggesting that 30% of the patients are cured of moderate to severe acute GVHD, many of these patients were transplanted prior to the availability of cyclosporine. GVHD prophylaxis for these patients consisted predominantly of methotrexate-based regimens, either alone or in conjunction with anti-thymocyte globulin (ATG), and prednisone or ex vivo T-cell depletion. It appears that the more recent patients transplanted with cyclosporine-based prophylactic regimens and who develop GVHD do not respond as well to the various treatments.

The Seattle group also reported a retrospective analysis of therapy for acute GVHD for patients who failed primary treatment.[6] Four hundred twenty-seven patients were identified. The majority of the patients had a rash (75%), with liver dysfunction as the second most common manifestation (59%) and gut difficulties as the third in 53% of the patients. Secondary treatment consisted of glucocorticoids in the majority of the patients (n=249), cyclosporine (n=80), anti-thymocyte globulin (n=214) or monoclonal antibody (n=19). Most patients received single treatments, however, 37 received a combination of these single agents. Improvement or resolution of GVHD in the respective organs was seen in 45% of the patients with skin disease, 25% of the patients with liver disease and 35% of the patients with gut disease. Forty percent of the patients showed some response. The highest complete response rate was seen when GVHD recurred during the taper phase of primary glucocorticoid treatment. Increasing the dose of glucocorticoids seemed to allow for a second complete response. Severe dysfunction in the skin, liver or gut at the beginning of treatment was associated with lower incidence of response or improvement in outcome. Although increasing the dose of glucocorticoids appeared to represent the most effective therapy or strategy when GVHD recurred during the taper phase or primary treatment, less than half the patients showed a durable overall improvement. These results suggest that the potential efficacy of immunosuppressive agents can be assessed meaningfully in patients who have not responded adequately to primary treatment and that more effective treatments are needed.

## ANTI-THYMOCYTE GLOBULIN

The Seattle transplant team reported its results using anti-thymocyte globulin (ATG) among 60 patients with grade II GVHD: 36 improved, 12 did not improve and 12 had progressive disease.[7] A subsequent randomized trial compared ATG on alternative days for six doses and prednisolone, 200 mg/kg/day for 10 days.[8] More responses were seen in the steroid group although the difference was not significant. All organ systems appeared to respond in the steroid group whereas ATG-treated patients experienced only few and incomplete responses in the GI tract and liver. Another study investigated the combination of ATG and cyclosporine.[9] Some of these patients also received methylprednisolone. Survival was low in patients receiving the triple immunosuppression of cyclosporine, ATG and methylprednisolone. The lower survival was due mostly to infectious complications. Untoward effects of ATG included hemolytic anemia, severe thrombocytopenia, neutropenia, fever, chills, polyarthritis, myalgias, nausea, vomiting, urticaria and serum sickness.

## CYCLOSPORINE

Although cyclosporine has been used for treatment of graft-versus-host disease, currently its primary function is in the prophylaxis of acute GVHD. Once a patient fails prophylaxis, the only treatment option is to increase the dose of cyclosporine. Unfortunately, there does not appear to be clear dose response phenomena, and it is not easy to dose escalate cyclosporine because of its propensity to cause renal dysfunction.

## MONOCLONAL ANTIBODIES

Monoclonal antibody OKT3 was first shown to be effective in treating recipients with renal transplant rejection. Since treatment with monoclonal antibody OKT3, specific for the CD3 complex instead of the T-cell antigen receptor, can reverse or cure rejection of human renal allografts, use of OKT3 has been attempted for the treatment of GVHD. A pilot trial in eight allogeneic recipients with grade II or IV acute GVHD showed response in six patients, especially those with very minimal disease.[10] In a second study of ten patients with grade III-IV acute GVHD who were resistant to cyclosporine, methylprednisolone, OKT3 induced complete responses in five and partial responses in four patients. However, acute GVHD recurred frequently.[11] The efficacy of anti-CD3 antibodies for the treatment of patients with GVHD has not been established. The dose limiting side effect results from T-cell activation induced by some of the anti-CD3 antibodies in vivo. This has discouraged further use of this monoclonal antibody. A different approach was used in a phase I/II study with an anti-CD3 antibody called BC3.[12] This is an anti-CD3 antibody that cannot cross-link CD3 with Fc receptors on accessory cells. Thus, it cannot induce T-cell proliferation. BC3 is a murine IgG2b that reacts with the CD3 complex but does not interact well with Fc receptors on human monocytes. Therefore, BC3 does not activate proliferation of T lymphocytes. Seventeen patients were enrolled in this study and five patients achieved a complete resolution of GVHD. Eight patients had partial improvement, two patients had no change and two patients had progression. Eight of the 13 patients had sustained responses. Interestingly, the administration of this non-mitogenic anti-CD3 antibody did not depend on depletion of the circulating T cells. The absolute count of peripheral blood lymphocytes decreased transiently but returned to baseline within 22 hours after the first infusion. The mechanism of action of this antibody therefore is related to some form of immunosuppression through modulation of T-cell function. Unfortunately, the use of OKT3 or anti-CD3 monoclonal antibodies results in lymphoproliferative syndrome from polyclonal proliferation of B cells infected with the Epstein-Barr virus. This is frequently a fatal complication of the immunodeficiency state after transplantation. Clearly, further clinical trials are necessary to establish the importance of these newer agents in the treatment of acute GVHD. In another trial by the Seattle team, four different IgG2a monoclonal antibodies designated 9.6, 35.1, 10.2 and 12.1 were given to 15 patients.[13] Six of 10 patients had at least partial improvement in one organ system involved.

Another approach has been the use of anti-IL-2 receptor monoclonal antibody (B-B10, CD25) to treat patients with a steroid-resistant grade II-IV acute GVHD.[14] Twenty-three patients were treated. Monoclonal antibody was given at 5 mg/day for 10 days and another five doses every other day. There was an 84% overall response rate (65% complete, 19% partial). Responses seem most likely with early treatment.

These early trials of an anti-IL-2 receptor monoclonal antibody (B-B10) for the treatment of acute GVHD showed promising results.[16] In a multi-center pilot study, 32 patients who experienced steroid-resistant acute GVHD were treated with this anti-IL-2 receptor monoclonal antibody. A full response of organ involvement was achieved in 22 patients (68.7%). Unfortunately, this study did not state whether these responses were durable. A follow-up study of 58 patients reported that 26 out of 58 (44.8%) were alive between 240 and 900 days after GVHD treatment with B-B10.[17] The significant factors associated with GVHD response were (1) the delay between the onset of GVHD and B-B10 treatment (p=.03), (2) the recurrence of liver involvement (patients without liver disease had a significantly higher response rate [p<0.01]) and (3) pretreatment level serum soluble CD8 antigen, where elevated or increasing levels of soluble CD8 were negatively correlated with response to the monoclonal antibody. Although the response rate was gratifying, the GVHD recurrence rate remained quite high at 41%. However, there was a significant survival advantage for those who responded to treatment with B-B10. Preliminary results, also for using the antibody for the prevention of acute GVHD, showed no problem with lack of engraftment and an apparent prevention of acute GVHD. Serial determination of soluble CD8, soluble IL-2 receptors and TNF-α suggests that serial measurements could provide valuable predictive information for the responsiveness of patients with acute GVHD to anti-IL-2 receptor monoclonal antibodies.[18]

Monoclonal antibody against TNF-α is another method for the treatment of severe acute GVHD. A monoclonal anti-TNF-α, termed B-C7, has been used to treat patients suffering from grade III-IV acute GVHD. Eighteen patients responded, 21% with a complete response and 61% with improvement. However, active GVHD appeared rapidly in eight patients. Only 22% of the patients were alive following treatment with anti-TNF.[19] More patients will need to be treated to extend these observations. This pilot study suggests that a monoclonal anti-TNF-α antibody may be of benefit to some patients with severe refractory acute GVHD but is ineffective in preventing GVHD recurrence in the majority of the patients.

In a multi-center pilot trial, 19 patients with severe GVHD refractory to conventional therapy and anti-IL-2 receptor antibodies received the antibody B-C7.[15] Ten patients were grafted from genotypically identical siblings, five from an HLA-mismatched family member and four from HLA-matched unrelated donors. No complete responses were observed, however, eight patients achieved a good partial response. Gut lesions responded the best, followed by skin and then liver. GVHD recurred when treatment was discontinued. Three patients are alive following treatment with this monoclonal antibody.

Another approach has been to use Xomazyme.[20] Thirty-four patients with moderate to severe steroid-resistant acute GVHD were treated with Xomazyme. Seventy-two percent responded in at least one organ and another 16% had stable disease. However, GVHD recurrence was frequent. Major difficulties with using murine monoclonal antibody include febrile reactions, fluctuation in blood counts and, most importantly, B-cell lymphoproliferative disorders that may lead to death in a large number of patients. Flu-like symptoms including fever, tremors, lethargy, anorexia, myalgias and arthralgias were observed with ricin-A immunoconjugants.

An alternative treatment strategy for acute GVHD was attempted with an anti-Ly1 monoclonal antibody conjugated to yttrium-90 in a murine model.[21] This approach was based on data showing that the cells responsible for GVHD induction expressed Ly1 on the cell surface. This Ly1 antigen is homologous to the CD5 structure in humans. Improved survival was found in mice who had established GVHD induced across major histocompatibility barrier. The therapeutic window obtained with yttrium-90 anti-Ly1 treatment was narrow. In addition, hematological analysis showed a reduction in total white blood cell count as well as absolute lymphocyte count and absolute neutrophil numbers. This myelosuppression recovered following cessation of treatment.

## OTHER IMMUNOSUPPRESSIVE DRUGS

Thalidomide has been used for the treatment of rodent models with GVHD.[22] In this rat model, thalidomide was effective for both the prevention and treatment of GVHD. One significant disadvantage for use in humans is the erratic absorption following oral administration.

## UNRELATED DONOR BMT

Treatment for acute GVHD following unrelated donor marrow transplantation suggests that more aggressive therapies are warranted in these patients.[23] Standard treatment with prednisone and ATG appears to be ineffective. When comparing with histocompatible sibling BMT, the Minnesota group reported that therapy for acute GVHD is associated with a 41% complete and continuing response rate.[5] But, of the 42 patients who underwent treatment with prednisone and ATG, only 9 achieved a complete and continuous response of acute GVHD by day +100 (21%). This increase in GVHD following unrelated donor BMT is due to the greater histocompatibility differences between the donor and recipient.

There is some suggestion that acute GVHD following a matched unrelated donor transplantation may respond to very high doses of methylprednisolone. In one small series of eight patients, high-dose methylprednisolone, 5 mg/kg/day for four days, and dose escalation to 10 mg/kg/day for nonresponders as initial therapy for acute GVHD was associated with a response in a majority of the patients.[24] Unfortunately, high-dose methylprednisolone was associated with severe, life-threatening, infectious complications.

## REFERENCES

1. Bagacilupo A, van Lint MT, Frassoni F et al. High dose bolus methylprednisolone for the treatment of acute graft-versus-host disease. Blut 1983; 46: 125.

2. Kanojia M, Anagnostou AA, Zander AR et al. High-dose methylprednisolone treatment for acute graft-versus-host disease after bone marrow transplantation in adults. Transplantation 1984; 37: 246.

3. Neudorf S, Filipovich A, Ramsay N, Kersey J. Prevention and treatment of acute graft-versus-host disease. Sem Hematol 1984; 21: 91.

4. Storb R, Deeg HJ, Whitehead J et al. Methotrexate and cyclosporine compared with cyclosporine alone for prophylaxis of acute graft-versus-host disease after marrow transplantation for leukemia. N Engl J Med 1986; 314: 729.

5. Weisdorf D, Haake R, Blazar et al. Treatment of moderate/severe acute graft-versus-host disease after allogeneic bone marrow transplantation: An analysis of clinical risk factors and outcome. Blood 1990; 75: 1024.

6. Martin P, Schoch G, Fisher L et al. A retrospective analysis of therapy for acute graft-versus-host disease: Secondary treatment. Blood 1991; 77: 1821.

7. Storb R, Gluckman RE, Thomas ED et al. Treatment of established human graft-versus-host disease by antithymocyte globulin. Blood 1974; 44: 57.

8. Doney K, Weiden PL, Storb R, Thomas ED. Treatment of graft-versus-host disease in human allogeneic marrow graft recipients: A randomized trial comparing antithymocyte globulin and corticosteroids. Am J Hematol 1981; 11: 1.

9. Deeg H, Loughran TP Jr, Storb R et al. Treatment of human acute graft-versus-host disease with anti-thymocyte globulin and cyclosporine with or without methylprednisolone. Transplantation 1985; 401: 162.

10. Gratama J, Jansen J, Lopovich RA, Tanke HJ, Goldstein G, Zwaan FE. Treatment of acute graft-versus-host disease with monoclonal antibody OKT3. Transplantation 1984; 38:469.

11. Gluckman E, Devergie A, Varin F, Rabian C, D'Agay MF, Benbunan M. Treatment of steroid resistant severe acute graft-versus-host disease with a monoclonal pan T OKT3 antibody. Exp Hematol 1984; 12: 66.

12. Anasetti C, Martin PJ, Storb R et al. Treatment of acute graft-versus-host disease with a nonmitogenic anti-CD3 monoclonal antibody. Transplantation 1992; 54: 844.

13. Martin P, Remlinger K, Hansen JA et al. Murine monoclonal anti-T-cell antbodies for treatment of refractory acute graft-versus-host disease. Transplant Proc 1984; 16: 1494.

14. Herve P, Wijdenes J, Bergerat JP et al. Treatment of corticosteroid resistant acute graft-versus-host disease by in vivo administration of anti-interleukin-2 receptor monoclonal antibody (B-B10). Blood 1990; 75: 1017.

15. Herve P, Flesch M, Tiberghien P et al. Phase I-II trail of a monoclonal anti-tumor necrosis factor α antibody for the treatment of refractory severe acute graft-versus-host disease. Blood 1992; 79: 3362.

16. Wijdenes J, Beliard R, Muot S, Herve P, Peters A. A semi-pharmaceutical approach for the preparation of an anti-IL2 receptor monoclonal antibody in the treatment of acute GVHD in a multicentric study. Develop Biol Stnd 1990; 71: 103.

17. Herve P, Bordigoni P, Cahn JY et al. Use of monoclonal antibodies in vivo as a therapeutic strategy for acute GvHD in matched and mismatched bone marrow transplantation. Transpl Proc 1991; 23: 1692.

18. Tiberghien P, Racadot E, Lioure B et al. Soluble CD8; IL-2 receptor, and tumor necrosis factor-alpha levels in steroid-resistant acute graft-versus-host disease. Transplantation 1991; 52: 475.

19. Herve P. Perspectives in the prevention and treatment of acute graft-versus-host disease. Bone Marrow Transpl 1991; 7 Suppl: 117.

20. Byers V, Henslee PJ, Kernan NA et al. Use of anti-pan T-lymphocyte ricin A chain immunotoxin in steroid-resistant acute graft-versus-host disease. Blood 1990; 75: 1426.

21. Vallera D, Schmidberger H, Buchsbaum DJ, Everson P, Snover DC, Blazer BR. Radiotherapy in mice with Yttrium-90-labeled anti-Ly1 monoclonal antibody: Therapy of established graft-versus-host disease induced across the major histocompatibility barrier. Cancer Res 1991; 51: 1891.

22. Vogelsang G, Taylor S, Gordon G, Hess AD. Thalidomide, a potent agent for the treatment of graft-versus-host disease. Transplant Proc 1986; 18: 904.

23. Roy J, McGlave PB, Filipovich AH et al. Acute graft-versus-host disease following unrelated donor marrow transplantation:Failure of conventional therapy. Bone Marrow Transplant 1992; 10: 77.

24. Oblon D, Felker D, Coyle K, Myers L. High-dose methylprednisolone therapy for acute graft-versus-host disease associated with matched unrelated donor bone marrow transplantation. Bone Marrow Transplant 1992; 10: 355.

# CHAPTER 10

# CHRONIC GVHD

## INTRODUCTION

Graft-versus-host disease has historically been divided into acute and chronic phase. The acute phase is, by definition, GVHD occurring within the first 100 days following allogeneic bone marrow grafting. Chronic graft-versus-host disease is defined as GVHD occurring after the first 100 days following allogeneic BMT. Chronic GVHD is the single major determinant of long-term outcome and quality of life following BMT. The morbidity and mortality associated with chronic GVHD remains a serious and very important problem. Chronic GVHD involves target tissues which are different from sites affected by acute GVHD. Moreover, histologic features show distinct differences between acute and chronic GVHD. Chronic GVHD appears to be associated more with an autoimmune phenomena including autoantibody formation. Aspects of chronic GVHD mimic systemic lupus erythematosus, scleroderma, progressive systemic sclerosis, lichen planus, sicca syndrome, eosinophilic fasciatis, rheumatoid arthritis and primary biliary sclerosis.[1] None of these collagen vascular diseases explain all the spectrum observed for chronic GVHD. Renal and CNS involvement are rarely seen in chronic GVHD. Chronic GVHD can be defined as limited or extensive, depending on the clinical presentation in patients (Table 10.1).

Chronic GVHD has a secondary effect, as it leads to a marked immunodeficiency in these patients. Chronic GVHD, in and of itself, is immunosuppressive and following the treatment for chronic GVHD, usually

---

*Table 10.1. Chronic GVHD grades*

| | |
|---|---|
| Limited: | Disease localized only to skin or hepatic involvement |
| Extensive: | 1. Generalized skin involvement |
| | 2. Limited skin involvement or hepatic involvement and |
| |     a. liver histology showing chronic progressive hepatits, bridging necrosis or cirrhosis |
| |     b. eye involvement (Schirmer's test with <5mm wetting) |
| |     c. involvement of minor salivary glands or oral mucosa |
| |     d. involvement of any other organ |

---

involving more immunosuppressive agents, results in increased immunosuppression. Chronic GVHD also causes a delay in the recovery of immune function. Patients remain immunodeficient as long as the disease is active.[2] T- and B-lymphocyte control remains dysregulated.[3] Recurrent infectious processes may occur in up to 100% of these patients under prolonged observation. These infectious complications account for the bulk of morbidity and mortality associated with chronic GVHD.

## LABORATORY DATA

### AUTOANTIBODIES

The autoantibodies in chronic GVHD are similar to those found in systemic lupus erythematosus or other collagen vascular diseases. These autoantibodies are usually anti-nuclear antibodies and their appearance coincides with early clinical symptoms of chronic GVHD.[4] The autoantibodies react with the nucleoli rather than with antigens such as Sm, nuclear RNPs, Ro/SSB, La/SSB and the scleroderma 70 antigen which are usually found in other autoimmune diseases. These autoantibodies may even lead to membranous nephropathy.[5] Anti-mitochondrial antibodies are also related to chronic GVHD.[6] The presence of these autoantibodies suggests that there might be a close relationship between chronic GVHD and primary biliary cirrhosis (also associated with elevated anti-mitochondrial antibodies), and that there might be a related pathologic event(s). One such possibility is endotoxin from gram-negative gut organisms. Endotoxin stimulates lymphocytes and macrophages resulting in elevated levels of IL-1, TNF and interferon-$\gamma$. These cytokines may lead to elevated MHC class II expression and further T-cell activation with enhanced GVHD or de novo GVHD.

Autoantibodies reacting to self-antigens involved in organ-specific autoimmunity, such as thyroglobulin, do not normally develop. One pathological alteration of chronic GVHD is hyperplasia of host B cells with production of lupus-like autoantibodies. This hyperstimulation of host B cells was demonstrated to be induced, and the response maintained by, alloreactive donor T cells.[7] This conclusion is supported by a murine model where (a) removal of T cells results in a drop in the titers of autoantibodies, (b) persistence of donor T cells in the host and (c) adoptive transfer of mice affected with GVHD into normal secondary recipients induced signs of chronic GVHD.

### ANTIBODIES

Investigators demonstrated that IgA deficiency occurs in many patients following allogeneic BMT.[8,9] This deficiency seems to be related to the development of acute and chronic GVHD.[10] There is a significant association between chronic GVHD and low serum IgA levels one to two years after BMT.[11] Chronic GVHD does not however appear to play an independent role in the development of IgA deficiency since all patients who developed chronic GVHD de novo had normal IgA levels at all times. In chronic GVHD, it is thought that helper T cells react against MHC incompatibility and generate excessive help. This excessive help activates a subpopulation of self-reactive B cells. By studying the various allotypes of autoantibody production in a murine model, Morris et al suggest that host B cells play a unique role in this GVHD autoimmune syndrome.[12] These B cells are regulated in an allotype-specific manner, some of which are presumably regulated by interactions with donor T cells.

## T Cells

Patients with chronic GVHD have an increase in nonspecific suppressor T cells which play an important role in the disease process. These cells can suppress T-cell proliferation and polyclonal immunoglobulin synthesis induced by various antigens.[3,13,14] Immunophenotyping of patients with chronic GVHD found an increase in CD8+ lymphocytes.[15] Analysis of these CD8+ cells revealed an increase in CD8+ CD11+(cells which suppress mitogen induced T-cell proliferation), CD8+ CD11- (precursor CTLs), and CD8+Leu7+ cells. The increase in these cells correlated closely with clinical evidence of disease.

## Cytokines

Another way to detect the presence of GVHD is by measurement of interleukin-3 (IL-3) which can serve as an indicator of the disease activity in GVHD.[16] IL-3 is a major regulator of myeloid cell growth and is involved in the regulation of immune cells. IL-3 is primarily produced by activated T cells, NK cells and mast cells. IL-3 is measured by enzyme-linked immunosorbents. Measurable levels of IL-3 were detected in a significant subgroup of patients suffering from extensive chronic GVHD. These levels were not associated with other pathologic conditions such as infectious diseases. However, IL-3 was not detectable prior to the onset of severe chronic GVHD. IL-3 was also detectable in a small subgroup of patients suffering from acute GVHD. These data suggest that IL-3 can be measurable in patients suffering from GVHD.

# CLINICAL MANIFESTATIONS OF CHRONIC GVHD

## Skin

The most frequent feature of chronic GVHD involves the skin. The pathological lesions resemble lichen planus and scleroderma. Two forms of expression of this disease are described. The first type is a generalized form where there is hyperkeratosis and epidermal hypertrophy. A lichenoid reaction is seen at the basal layer. In a late phase, the dermis becomes atrophic and the inflammatory changes are less striking. The ridges become absent and the dermal-epidermal junction becomes straightened and obliterated. Fibrosis can be observed throughout the dermis and the adnexal structures. The second form is localized skin involvement with epidermal atrophy and dense focal dermal fibrosis in the absence of significant inflammation. This type of chronic GVHD more closely resembles that of morphea and lupus. There is damage to the basal lamina, the basal cell layer and the spinous layer similar to lesions seen in the lichen planus.[17] The onset of skin involvement may be generalized erythema with plaques and waves of desquamation with continued underlying erythema. Not infrequently, patients will give a history of photoactivation. UV radiation may damage superficial epidermal cells leading to increased antigen expression and increased cytokine release with the resultant expression of chronic GVHD. The skin shows alternating areas of hyper- and hypopigmentation. Without effective treatment, the skin may become progressively indurated and fixed to the underlying fascia. The epidermis becomes significantly atrophic with prominent poikiloderma. Some patients have localized lesions resembling that of morphea. The end result, without specific treatment, is that of hyperpigmentation or hypopigmentation, hide-like skin and joint contractures not unlike that seen with scleroderma.[18,19]

## LIVER

Chronic liver GVHD is also observed very frequently in patients. A biopsy specimen may show lobular hepatitis, chronic persistent hepatitis or chronic active hepatitis.[20] There is a reduction or absence of small bile ducts with cholestasis. The pathophysiology of chronic GVHD suggests primary biliary sclerosis.[21] There appears to be biliary cell necrosis and thickening of the bile duct basement membranes. Hepatic function tests show a predominant cholestatic picture. The degree of hyperbilirubinemia may not reflect the ultimate outcome. Patients may have persistent hyperbilirubinemia for many years before improvement or severe hepatic failure develops.

Liver injury and murine chronic GVHD to minor histocompatibility antigens is characterized by mononuclear cell infiltration and necrosis of interlobular bile ducts.[22] This is similar to what occurs in human GVHD, late liver transplant rejection and primary biliary sclerosis. Isolation of mononuclear inflammatory cells from the liver during chronic GVHD showed a progressive increase in homing of these mononuclear cells to the liver of recipient mice. Autoradiographs determined the intrahepatic sites at which chronic GVHD liver mononuclear cells accumulate after injection, and demonstrated that these mononuclear cells accumulate preferentially in the hepatic portal spaces in close proximity to the interlobular bile ducts. These results suggest that hepatic homing by such mononuclear cells is specific for minor histocompatibility antigens expressed on the host biliary epithelial cells. Thus, the bile duct obstruction is mediated by mononuclear cells which appear to be sensitized to minor histocompatibility antigens expressed in the host biliary epithelial cells.

## GASTROINTESTINAL TRACT

The gut is another frequent site of GVHD. The oral mucosa is involved in the majority of patients with extensive GVHD.[18,23] Patients develop dryness with pain secondary to ulceration. Erythema with lichenoid lesions of the buccal and labial mucosa was found to correlate with chronic GVHD.[24] Increasing oral symptoms, either that of increasing ulceration or pain, seem to be associated with progression of GVHD. The esophagus is also involved in chronic GVHD. Patients may develop dysphagia, painful ulcers and indolent weight loss. A radiograph may include findings such as webs, ring-like narrowing and tapering structure of the mid and upper esophagus.[25] The small bowel and the colon may also be involved in chronic GVHD. Patients may develop chronic diarrhea, malabsorption, fibrosis of the submucosa and sclerosis of the intestine.

## LUNG

Obstructive lung disease may develop in patients with chronic GVHD and appears to be refractory to therapy.[26] Bronchiolitis obliterans occasionally with organizing pneumonia may be seen.[27-30] The possible etiologies of bronchiolitis obliterans are broad and include pulmonary infections (especially viral or mycoplasma), irradiation injury, toxic inhalants, connective tissue diseases and pulmonary alveolar proteinosis. Clinically, patients present with dyspnea and a nonproductive cough. Bronchiolitis obliterans causes destruction of small airways. Fibrous obliteration of the lumen and the bronchioles is observed in the histology. This granulation tissue often extends into the alveolar ducts. It is unclear, however, whether the lungs are a primary or secondary target in chronic GVHD. The incidence of bronchiolitis obliterans seems to be associated with chronic GVHD and a decreased serum IgG.[31] These results suggest that possible use of IVIg in conjunction with early detection may be beneficial for these patients. Otherwise, bronchiolitis obliterans usually leads to progressive respiratory failure.

## OTHER MANIFESTATIONS

Gynecological manifestations in GVHD have also been observed. These include vaginal inflammation, sicca syndrome and vaginal stenosis.[32,33] Other manifestations of chronic GVHD include polymyositis, which responds well to steroid therapy.[34] Myasthenia gravis has also been associated with chronic GVHD.[35] Symptoms appear usually during the time corticosteroids are being tapered. Membranous nephropathy has also been associated with chronic GVHD, similar to that observed in the murine model.[5]

Various antibodies were screened in 53 long-term survivors after allogeneic bone marrow transplantation.[36] Among these patients, 40 displayed chronic graft-versus-host disease. The auto antibodies were found as follows: anti-nuclear antibody (62.2%), anti-smooth muscle (49%), anti-mitochondria (11.3%), anti-liver kidney microsome (5.6%) and anti-epidermal antibodies (11.3%). Screening for native anti-DNA, anti-extractable nuclear antigen, anti-centromere and anti-salivary gland duct antibodies was negative. The presence or absence of acute GVHD made no difference in the frequency of auto antibodies. No correlation was evident between cutaneous or hepatic involvement, sicca syndrome, scleroderma status and autoantibodies. Despite the clinical features mimicking collagen vascular disease, the biological autoimmune profile of GVHD was different. These data suggest that chronic GVHD may have a different pathophysiologic mechanism.

The occurrence of autoantibodies in relation to chronic GVHD has also been studied in children.[37] Seventeen of 40 patients developed auto antibodies to thyroid microsomes, compared to none of 46 control children of similar age. The presence of these autoantibodies was strongly associated with the presence of chronic GVHD. Other antibodies strongly correlated with the occurrence of chronic GVHD were IgG antibodies to the cytoplasm of squamous epithelial cells. Antibodies to nuclei, smooth muscle and gastric parietal cells were present but did not correlate with the presence of chronic GVHD. This study suggests that antibodies to thyroid antigens and to the cytoplasm of squamous epithelial cells may be a useful marker for chronic GVHD.

## GRADING

Chronic GVHD may be graded as limited where the disease is either localized to skin involvement only or to hepatic dysfunction. Alternatively, chronic GVHD may present as extensive disease with generalized or localized skin involvement and hepatic dysfunction plus (1) liver histology showing chronic progressive hepatitis; bridging necrosis or cirrhosis, (2) involvement of eye—Schirmer's test with less than 5 mm wetting, (3) involvement of minor salivary glands, oral mucosa demonstrated on labial or mucosal biopsy specimen or (4) involvement of any other target organ. Usually, a 3 mm punch biopsy is used to secure full dermal thickness specimen of the skin including a portion of subcutaneous fat. A biopsy of sun exposed forearm areas can show diagnostic changes, even in the absence of a rash. Oral biopsies are also very effective in detecting the presence of chronic GVHD.

Chronic GVHD occurs in approximately 50% of long-term survivors of HLA identical sibling transplants.[38] A survey was conducted to assess the reproducibility among clinicians to determine the degree of concordance among bone marrow transplant physicians in the diagnosis, grading and treatment of chronic GVHD. Clinical case reports were composed based on patients treated at St. Vincent's Hospital in Sydney, Australia. Questionnaires were mailed to 160 bone marrow transplant centers worldwide. There was moderate to high concordance for the diagnosis, grading and treatment of chronic GVHD. Major disagreements were observed in the diagnosis of uncommon manifestations of chronic GVHD, interpretation of symptoms which occur less than two months after transplantation, interpretation of persistent stable symptoms and in deciding whether to treat chronic GVHD limited to skin. One interesting observation was that time of onset is an important clinical feature for some, but not all, transplanters in establishing diagnosis of chronic GVHD. Thus, these results point to potential problems in interpreting certain clinical trials to prevent or treat chronic GVHD. The results demonstrate that the diagnostic grading criteria showed little disagreement between transplant centers. However, consistency in grading the severity of the symptoms may be improved by using, for example, the Karnofsky performance status to differentiate between limited versus extensive chronic GVHD.

Patients who have limited disease have a favorable prognosis even without therapy. Patients with extensive, particularly multi-organ disease, have an unfavorable natural history. Approximately 50% of patients will develop chronic GVHD at some point after the first 100 days. The known risk factors for the development of chronic GVHD are listed in Table 10.2.

### Table 10.2. Risk factors of the occurrence of chronic GVHD

Degree of HLA matching
Age (donor and recipient)
Subacute GVHD detected by skin biopsy
Subacute GVHD detected by buccal mucosal biopsy
History of grade II-IV acute GVHD
Splenectomy
Cytomegalovirus seropositivity (donor and recipient)

## RISK FACTORS

Some variability will depend on the degree of HLA matching. Data from Seattle in 1,431 patients with hematological malignancies showed a significant increase in chronic GVHD in patients receiving marrow from HLA identical family members, nonidentical family members or unrelated donors (33% versus 49% versus 64%, respectively).[39] The median day of onset of GVHD was earlier in the mismatched patients. Very few patients developed chronic GVHD more than 500 days after transplantation. Another factor that may be predictive of chronic GVHD is age. The probability of developing chronic GVHD increases significantly in older bone marrow recipients. Additional predictive factors for developing chronic GVHD are prior acute GVHD and administration of unirradiated donor buffy code transfusions.[18,40] Other predictive factors include second bone marrow infusions, preceding herpes virus infection and absence of blood transfusions given shortly before transplantation.[41,42] There is evidence in murine models suggesting that non-H-2 factors exert a major influence in susceptibility for renal involvement in murine chronic graft-versus-host disease.[43]

Another study was conducted in 169 patients, with a number of screening studies performed between 71 to 121 days after allogeneic marrow grafting to detect the development of chronic GVHD. Group 1 patients were asymptomatic with a normal physical examination at the time of screening and had not developed chronic GVHD. Group 2 patients had signs or symptoms of chronic GVHD at the time of testing and group 3 patients had no initial clinical evidence of GVHD but later developed clinical chronic GVHD. Seventeen clinical laboratory factors were evaluated and screened to accurately predict development of subsequent chronic GVHD. Multivariant analyses of these 17 factors showed several to have independent predictive value.[44] Predictive factors included histological finding of GVHD in a skin biopsy and history of grade II-IV acute GVHD. Oral biopsy results were not included in the first model since only half of the patients had oral biopsies. When oral biopsies were included, the independent risk factors then included histological finding of GVHD in the skin biopsy and low numbers of immunoglobulin A-bearing plasma cells detected by direct immunofluorescence in salivary gland areas on oral biopsy. The ability to predict the possible occurrence of subsequent chronic GVHD is important because immunosuppressive therapy has greatly decreased the morbidity and mortality associated with chronic GVHD. Alternatively, patients who may never develop GVHD do not need continued immunosuppressive therapy. Initial studies suggest that early use of combination immunosuppressive therapy is effective in decreasing morbidity associated with chronic GVHD.[18] A prospective randomized clinical trial begun in 1980 demonstrated the efficacy of early treatment with steroid therapy in patients with extensive chronic GVHD.[45] Some patients in this trial had positive screening tests without symptoms or signs of clinically active chronic GVHD, i.e., subclinical extensive chronic GVHD. It was hoped that treatment of these patients before clinical manifestation of disease would prevent the clinical progression of extensive chronic GVHD. Unfortunately, more than 70% of patients with subclinical disease progressed to clinical chronic GVHD despite immunosuppressive therapy. Moreover, in patients in whom chronic GVHD remained subclinical, there was a statistically significant increased probability of relapse of malignant disease.

A separate study from Johns Hopkins University Medical Center also assessed the value of the predictors of death from chronic GVHD after bone marrow transplantation.[46] This study evaluated not only the development of extensive chronic GVHD but the relative risk of death from chronic GVHD. Limited involvement has been associated with a good prognosis.[20] The clinical manifestation has been an important determinant of outcome. Patients with progressive disease have a worse outcome than patients with other modes of presentation. Thrombocytopenia has also been reported to be a poor prognostic factor[45] and the type of treatment was reported as a determinant of outcome.[47] The study from Johns Hopkins, however, evaluated what baseline factors at the time of onset of chronic GVHD would predict survival from chronic GVHD. In this study of 85 patients with chronic GVHD, several baseline factors emerged as independent predictors of death: progressive presentation (chronic GVHD following acute GVHD without resolution of acute GVHD), lichenoid changes on the skin histology and elevation of serum bilirubin >1.2 mg/dL. Actuarial survival of patients with none of these risk factors was 70% at six years compared to a projected six-year survival and only 20% for patients with a combination of two or more of these factors. Thirty-eight patients with one of these risk factors had a projected six-year survival of 43%. Identification of these baseline risk factors will facilitate future designs of chronic GVHD therapies with possible assignment of high risk patients to more aggressive and newer regimens.

A third large study on chronic GVHD was performed by the leukemia working party of European BMT centers.[42] In this study, 285 patients who survived more than three months were evaluated for the development of chronic GVHD. These patients were reported from 17 European bone marrow transplantation teams. The cumulative incidence of chronic GVHD was 32% two years after BMT. Chronic GVHD in a bivariate analysis had a statistically significant association with high donor and recipient age, splenectomy, chronic myeloid leukemia, a previous grade II-IV acute GVHD, pretransplant cytomegalovirus seropositivity in the recipients and the donor, and donor seropositivity to three or four herpes virus prior to BMT. In a multivariate analysis, the statistically significant factors associated with the development of chronic GVHD were combined recipient and donor CMV seropositivity prior to BMT, a previous grade II-IV acute GVHD and splenectomy. This was the first large study to conclude that CMV serology was statistically significant for the development of chronic GVHD, especially when both the donor and recipient were seropositive for CMV. Therefore, CMV immune donor cells may be triggered by latent CMV in the recipient and this may play a role in the development of chronic GVHD, possibly through release of specific cytokines. Several studies have reported a close correlation between acute and chronic GVHD.[18,46] Thus immune triggering of acute and chronic GVHD may be similar, even if the manifestations are different. The general effector mechanisms may be similar as well. The role of cytokines in the development of chronic GVHD has not been thoroughly investigated. It is likely that, although the clinical manifestations of these disease are different, similar cytokines may be involved with similar outcomes for the development of GVHD but possibly with different effector cells. The risk factors which have been associated with a poor outcome in chronic GVHD are listed in Table 10.3.

---

**Table 10.3. Risk factors for poor outcome in chronic GVHD**

Thrombocytopenia
Progressive presentation of GVHD
Lichenoid changes in skin histology
Elevated serum bilirubin > 1.2 mg/dl

---

## PREVENTION OF CHRONIC GVHD

Thymus tissue implants, thymic endothelial cells obtained from third party donors sharing one HLA-A and -B locus with the recipient or thymic hormone, thymosin fraction 5 and thymopentin have been given to recipients of HLA-matched sibling BMT in order to prevent chronic GVHD and to accelerate immunological reconstitution.[48] The clinical courses of 17 patients receiving thymic tissue and 18 patients receiving thymic hormones showed no difference in the incidence of chronic GVHD or immunologic recovery compared to concurrent or historical controls. Following this initial data, new manipulations were were performed to reduce the rejection of the thymic tissue graft by modifying the culture method to lower the number of lymphocytes in the thymic tissue implants. In spite of this modification, no benefit resulted from this manipulation.

## THERAPY OF CHRONIC GVHD

### PREDNISONE AND/OR CYCLOSPORINE

Sullivan and his colleagues in Seattle used the day-100 screening studito es, demonstrate that positive skin biopsy and history of prior acute GVHD independently predicted subsequent chronic GVHD. The study was designed to treat subclinical GVHD, i.e., patients who were asymptomatic with a positive random skin and oral biopsy showing histologic evidence of chronic GVHD. Immunosuppressive therapy was administered with patients being randomized to prednisone versus placebo versus prednisone and azathioprine. In this study, early treatment with prednisone alone in standard risk chronic GVHD was superior to treatment with a combination of prednisone and azathioprine.[45] In this same study, however, in high risk patients with persistent thrombocytopenia, prednisone alone resulted only in a 26% long-term survival. The same investigators later demonstrated that there was improved survival and a decrease in transplant-related mortality in patients with high risk chronic GVHD when treated with an alternating day regimen of cyclosporine and prednisone.[47] In that study, patients were placed on the regimen consisting of prednisone and cyclosporine given on alternate days. The five-year actuarial survival increased, from 26% with prednisone alone in the earlier study, to 51% in the subsequent study. There is an on-going randomized study comparing standard risk patients with platelet counts >100,000/μl to be randomized to receive either prednisone alone or cyclosporine and prednisone. Patients with high risk chronic GVHD are randomized to receive either cyclosporine alone or the cyclosporine and prednisone combination. Although an extensive amount of effort in trials has been placed on the prophylaxis and treatment of acute GVHD, the overall impact in disease-free survival is equally great in those patients suffering from chronic GVHD. Therefore, over the last several years, a significant amount of interest and effort has been placed in understanding, preventing and treating chronic GVHD.

## THALIDOMIDE

New agents have been entering clinical trials, including prospective randomized trials. One interesting drug which has been available for quite some time is thalidomide (N-phthalidoglutarimide). Thalidomide was introduced as a sleeping pill and showed a good activity combined with the absence of acute toxicity and side effects. Unfortunately, with long-term use, neurotoxicity became evident and the confirmed teratogenic activity led to the withdrawal of thalidomide from the market. It was found to be an immunosuppressant soon after its removal from the market.[49] The immunosuppressive problems with thalidomide have been known for over 20 years. It was first reported that patients with leprosy who received thalidomide as a sedative experienced relief of their symptoms of leprosy.[50] The use of thalidomide as an immunosuppressive has been reported for nearly all forms of autoimmune diseases. It has found a place in the primary mucocutaneous disorder including lepromatous leprosy, apthous stomatitis and discoid lupus erythematosus.[51] Because of teratogenic effects of thalidomide, its immunosuppressive properties have not been fully explored. In 1986, Vogelsang and the group at Johns Hopkins University reported on the use of thalidomide in the treatment of acute GVHD in a rat model for bone marrow transplantation. Animals which develop GVHD in this model demonstrate clinical characteristics similar to what is seen in patients developing this condition after allogeneic bone marrow transplantation. The animals receiving thalidomide had less toxicity and a higher response rate than animals receiving either azathioprine and prednisone or cyclosporine with or without prednisone. Subsequent data confirmed its value in chronic GVHD.[52,53] A study has been carried out at Johns Hopkins University treating 44 patients resulting in an overall response rate of 64%.[54] Survival was 76% among the patients receiving salvage therapy for refractory GVHD and 48% among those with high risk GVHD. These studies suggest the efficacy of thalidomide in treating established chronic GVHD. A phase I-II trial with thalidomide in patients with refractory GVHD or high risk GVHD has also been performed suggesting that it has some efficacy in the treatment of established chronic GVHD. Eighteen patients were treated at the City of Hope National Medical Center. Ten out of the 18 responded with improvement within two months, including 6 of 7 patients with primary oral manifestation of the disease, 2 of 4 patients with primary skin manifestation, 2 of 3 patients with pulmonary manifestation and 1 patient with liver disease.[55] Patients who evolved from severe acute GVHD did not respond to the drug. Other than sedation and constipation, the therapy was well-tolerated with only one patient requiring discontinuation. We have also used thalidomide in patients who developed overt chronic GVHD while on a cyclosporine and prednisone taper. The overall complete response rate has been approximately 20-25%. The differences in overall response rate may be related to standard versus high-risk characteristics and whether patients had de novo, rapidly progressive chronic GVHD, or had developed chronic GVHD while on immunosuppression.

## Psoralen Ultraviolet Irradiation

One other area of interest is psoralen ultraviolet irradiation (PUVA) treatment.[56-59] There has been an increased interest in the immunosuppressive effect of ultraviolet irradiation.[60] The proposed mechanism for PUVA is inhibition of DNA transcription and mitosis. Upon activation with ultraviolet A light, photoexcited psoralen covalently binds to one or both strands of DNA. The psoralen forms monoadducts or bifunctional adducts with intrastrand linkage between opposite DNA strands and therefore damages DNA. Psoralen can also damage mitochondria and therefore affect cell function. During PUVA treatment, the circulating lymphocytes are exposed to 1-5% of the skin surface radiation dose. This results in a decrease in the number and function of circulating lymphocytes. There is a decrease in T-cell proliferation, mitogen response and NK activity.[61] There may be UV-resistant antigen-presenting cells that activate suppressor pathways.[62] Ultraviolet radiation has also an effect on cytokine production, specifically in IL-1 and IL-2; however, these observations were made either in vitro or in psoriasis patients.[63] The results in patients after BMT may be different. A recent review of PUVA reported that 3 out of 11 patients achieved a complete remission of chronic GVHD.[64] Unfortunately, the efficacy of PUVA seems to be limited primarily to skin complications of chronic GVHD. Perhaps use of this modality earlier in the course of chronic GVHD may be more effective. There is data that ultraviolet irradiation may modulate MHC-alloreactive cytotoxic T-cell precursors that are involved in the onset of GVHD.[65]

## Specific Therapies

Since chronic GVHD affecting the liver is a cholestatic disease associated with jaundice and elevation of alkaline phosphatase similar to primary biliary cirrhosis, a trial was carried out to evaluate the effect of ursodeoxycholic acid treatment.[66] Ursodeoxycholic acid is a relatively nontoxic hydrophilic bile acid with a striking choleresis effect. When ursodeoxycholic acid was utilized for patients with chronic GVHD, patients improved with a 33% decrease in the bilirubin level compared to baseline (p<0.005), 32% decrease in alkaline phosphatase (p<0.038), and a 37% decrease in AST (p<0.007). The levels of these serum tests rose after discontinuation of the drug. One possibility for the mechanism of action is that ursodeoxycholic acid simply replaces the more hydrophobic detergent and toxic bile acids. A more intriguing possibility could be an effect on the immune system suggested by the disappearance of aberrant expression of HLA class I antigens on hepatocytes after ursodeoxycholic acid treatment of primary biliary cirrhosis.[67]

## Newer Agents

Newer agents have continued to be introduced including newer immunosuppressive agents such as FK506 and rapamycin both used in the treatment and prevention of GVHD.[68,69]

# CHRONIC GVHD AND AIDS

One of the more interesting and potentially fruitful avenues of investigation is the marked clinical immunological similarities between chronic GVHD and AIDS. The major features shared by chronic GVHD and HIV disease include activation of T cells, antigen-specific dysfunction, B-cell hyper-reactivity leading to hypergammaglobulinemia and autoreactive antibodies, change in $CD8^+$ T cells, suppressor cells selective for $CD4^+$ T cells, cyto-toxicity for autologous cells, skin lesions, GI disease, lymphadenopathy, opportunistic infection, high grade lymphomas, angiodysplastic-like lesions, and cytokine dysregulation including tumor necrosis factor and IL-6. One possibility for this similarity is that the HIV antigens may mimic allogeneic MHC molecules altering self-antigen-presenting cells or T cells such that they now appear as foreign cells.[70] In doing so, these HIV glycoproteins may stimulate alloreactive lymphocytes. This hypothesis is further strengthened by a clear difference in HLA haplotype between those patients who progress to AIDS gradually and those who progress at a slower rate or who have yet to progress.[71] Moreover, there seems to be a direct association between the rapid progression to AIDS and the extent of immune activation. This would suggest that the progression may be a genetically related aspect of viral infection.

## REFERENCES

1. Sullivan K. Acute and chronic graft-versus-host disease. Int J Cell Cloning 1986; 4:(1)42.

2. Witherspoon R, Storb R, Ochs HD et al. Recovery of antibody production in human allogeneic marrow graft recipients: Influence of time post-transplantation, the presence or absence of chronic graft-versus-host disease and antithymocyte globulin treatment. Blood 1981; 58: 360.

3. Lum L, Orcutt-Thordarson N, Seigneuret MC, Storb R. The regulation of Ig synthesis after marrow transplantation. IV. T4 and T8 subset function in patients with chronic graft-versus-host disease. J Immunol 1982; 129: 113.

4. Kier P, Penner E, Bakos S et al. Autoantibodies in chronic GVHD: High prevalence of antinucleolar antibodies. Bone Marrow Transpl 1990; 6: 93.

5. Barbara J, Thomas AC, Smith PS, Gillis D, Ho JOK, Woodroffe AJ. Membranous nephopathy with graft-versus-host disease in a bone marrow transplant recipient. Clinical Nephrology 1992; 37: 115.

6. Siegert W, Stemerowicz R, Hopf U. Antimitochondrial antibodies in patients with chronic graft-verus-host disease. Bone Marrow Transplant 1992; 10: 221.

7. Rozendahl L, Pals ST, Gleichmann E, Melief JM. Persistence of allospecific helper T cells is required for maintaining autoantibody formation in lupus-like graft-versus-host disease. Clin Exp Immunol 1990; 82: 527.

8. Elfenbein G, Anderson PN, Jumphrey RL et al. Immune system reconstitution following allogeneic bone marrow transplantation in man: A multiparameter analysis. Transplant Proc 1976; 8: 641.

9. Perreault C, Giasson M, Gyger M et al. Serum immunoglobulin levels following allogeneic bone marrow transplantation. Blut 1985; 51: 137.

10. Witherspoon R, Kopecky K, Storb R et al. Immunological recovery in 48 patients following syngeneic marrow transplantation for hematological malignancy. Transplantation 1982; 33: 143.

11. Abedi M, Hammarstrom L, Ringden O, Edvard Smith CI. Development of IgA deficiency after bone marrow transplantation. Transplantation 1990; 50: 415.

12. Morris S, Cheek RL, Cohen PL, Eisenberg RA. Allotype-specific immunoregulation of autoantibody production by host B cells in chronic graft-versus-host disease. J Immunol 1990; 144: 916.

13. Korsmeyer S, Elfenbein GJ, Goldman CK, Marshall SL, Waldmann TA. B cell, helper T-cell and suppressor T-cell abnormalities contribute to disordered immunoglobulin synthesis in patients following bone marrow transplantation. Transplantation 1982; 33: 184.

14. Tsoi M, Storb R, Hobbs et al. Nonspecific suppressor cells in patients with chronic graft-vs-host disease after marrow grafting. J Immunol 1979; 123: 1970.

15. Yabe H, Yabe M, Kato S, Kimura M, Iwaki K. Increased numbers of CD8+ CD11+, CD8+ CD11- and CD8+ Leu+ cells in patients with chronic graft-versus-host disease after allogeneic bone marrow transplantation. Bone Marrow Transplant 1990; 5: 295.

16. Valent P, Sillaber KCh, Scherrer R et al. Detection of circulating endogenous interleukin-3 in extensive chronic graft-versus-host disease. Bone Marrow Transpl 1992; 9: 331.

17. Gallucci B, Shulman HM, Sale GE, Lerner KG, Caldwell LE, Thomas ED. The ultrastructure of the human epidermis in chronic graft-versus-host disease. Am J Pathol 1979; 95: 643.

18. Sullivan K, Shulman HM, Storb R et al. Chronic graft-versus-host disease in 52 patients: Adverse natural course and successful treatment with combination immunosuppression. Blood 1981; 57: 267.

19. Shulman H, Sale GE, Lerner KG et al. Chronic cutaneous graft-versus-host disease in man. Am J Path 1978; 91: 545.

20. Schulman H, Sullivan KM, Weiden PL et al. Chronic graft-versus-host syndrome in man. A long-term clinicopathologic study of 20 Seattle patients. Am J Med 1980; 69: 204.

21. Epstein O, Thomas MC, Sherlock S. Primary biliary cirrhosis is a dry gland syndrome with features of chronic graft-versus-host disease. Lancet 1980; i: 1166.

22. Howell C, Yoder T, Claman HN, Vierling JM. Hepatic homing of mononuclear inflammatory cells isolated during murine chronic graft-versus-host disease. J Immunol 1989; 143: 476.

23. Schubert M, Sullivan KM. Recognition, incidence, and management of oral graft-versus-host disease. NCI Monogr 1990; 9: 135.

24. Schubert M, Sullivan KM, Morton TH et al. Oral manifestation of chronic graft-versus-host disease. Arch Intern Med 1984; 144: 1591.

25. McDonald G, Sullivan KM, Plumley TF. Radiographic features of esophageal involvement in chronic graft-versus-host disease. Am J Roent 1984; 142: 501.

26. Epler G. Bronchiolitis obliterans and airways obstruction associated with graft-versus-host disease. Clinics Chest Med 1988; 9: 551.

27. Rosenberg M, Vercellotti GM, Snover DC, Hurd D, McGlave P. Bronchiolitis obliterans after bone marrow transplantation. Am J Hematol 1985; 18: 325.

28. Wyatt S, Nunn P, Hows JM et al. Airway obstruction associated with graft-versus-host disease after bone marrow transplantation. Thorax 1984; 39: 887.

29. Ralph D, Springmeyer SC, Sullivan KM, Hackman RC, Storb R, Thomas ED. Rapidly progressive air-flow obstruction in marrow transplant recipients. Am Rev Respir Dis 1984; 129: 641.

30. Johnson F, Stokes DC, Ruggiero M, Dalla-Pozza L, Callihan TR. Chronic obstructive airways disease after bone marrow transplantation. J Pediat 1984; 105: 370.

31. Holland H, Wingard JR, Beschorner WE, Saral R, Santos GW. Bronchiolitis obliternas in bone marrow transplantation and its relationship to chronic graft-v-host disease and low serum IgG. Blood 1988; 72: 621.

32. Schubert M, Sullivan KM, Schubert MM et al. Gynecological abnormalities following allogeneic bone marrow transplantation. Bone Marrow Transplant 1990; 5: 425.

33. Corson S, Sullivan K, Batzer F, August C, Storb R, Thomas ED. Gynecological manifestations of chronic graft-versus-host disease. Obstet Gynecol 1982; 60: 488.

34. Reyes M, Noronha P, Thomas W Jr, Heredia R. Myositis of chronic graft-versus-host disease. Neurology 1983; 33: 1222.

35. Smith C, Aarli JA, Biberfeld P et al. Myasthenia gravis after bone marrow transplantation. Evidence for a donor origin. N Engl J Med 1983; 309: 1565.

36. Rouquette-Gally AM, Boyeldieu D, Prost, AC Gluckman E. Autoimmunity after allogeneic bone marrow transplantation. Transplantation 1988; 46: 238.

37. Lortan J, Rochfort NC, Tl-Tumi M, Vellodi A. Autoantibodies after bone marrow transplantation in children with genetic disorders: Relation to chronic graft-versus-host disease. Bone Marrow Transplant 1992; 9: 325.

38. Atkinson K, Horowitz MM, Gale RP et al. Consensus among bone marrow transplanters for diagnosis, grading and treatment of chronic graft-versus-host disease. Bone Marrow Transplant 1989; 4: 247.

39. Sullivan K, Agura E, Anasetti C et al. Chronic graft-versus-host disease and other late complications of bone marrow transplantation. Semin Hemat 1991; 28: 250.

40. Storb R, Prentice RL, Sullivan KM et al. Predictive factors in chronic graft-versus-host disease in patients with aplastic anemia treated by marrow transplantation from HLA-identical siblings. Ann Intern Med 1983; 98: 461.

41. Bolger G, Sullivan KM, Storb R et al. Second marrow infusion for poor graft function after allogeneic marrow transplantation. Bone Marrow Transplant 1986; 1: 21.

42. Bostrom L, Ringden O, Jacobsen N, Zwaan F, Nilsson B. A European multicenter study of chronic graft-versus-host disease. Transplantation 1990; 49: 1100.

43. Brujin J, Van Elven EH, Corver WE, Oudshoorn-Snoek M, Fleuren GJ. Genetics of experimental lupus nephritis: Non-H-2 factors determine susceptibility for renal involvement in murine chronic graft-versus-host disease. Clin Exp Immunol 1989; 76: 284.

44. Loughran T, Sullivan K, Morton T et al. Value of day 100 screening studies for predicting the development of chronic graft-versus-host disease after allogeneic bone marrow transplantation. Blood 1990; 76: 228.

45. Sullivan K, Witherspoon RP, Storb R et al. Prednisone and azathioprine compared with prednisone and placebo for treatment of chronic graft-v-host disease: Prognostic influence of prolonged thrombocytopenia after allogeneic marrow transplantation. Blood 1988; 72: 546.

46. Wingard J, Piantadosi S, Vogelsang GB et al. Predictors of death from chronic graft-versus-host disease after bone marrow transplantation. Blood 1989; 74: 1428.

47. Sullivan K, Witherspoon RP, Storb R et al. Alternating-day cyclosporine and prednisone for treatment of high-risk chronic graft-versus-host disease. Blood 1988; 72: 555.

48. Witherspoon R, Sullivan KM, Lum LG et al. Use of thymic grafts or thymic factors to augment immunologic recovery after bone marrow transplantation: brief report with 2 to 12 years' follow-up. Bone Marrow Transplant 1988; 3: 425.

49. Field E, Gibbs JE, Tucker DF, Hellmann K. Effect of thalidomide on the graft-versus-host reaction. Nature 1966; 211: 1308.

50. Sheskin J. Thalidomide in the treatment of lepra reactions. Clin Pharmac 1968; 6: 303.

51. Barnhill R, McDougall AC. Thalidomide: Use and possible mode of action in reactional lepromatous leprosy and in various other conditions. J Am Acad Dermatol 1982; 7: 317.

52. Vogelsang G, Wells MC, Santos GW, Chen TL, Hess AD. Combination low-dose thalidomide and cyclosporine prophylaxis for acute graft-versus-host disease in a rat mismatched model. Transpl Proc 1988; 20(Suppl 2): 226.

53. Heney D, Bailey CC, Lewis IJ. Thalidomide in the treatment of graft-versus-host disease. Biomed & Pharmacother 1990; 44: 199.

54. Vogelsang G, Farmer ER, Hess AD et al. Thalidomide for the treatment of chronic graft-versus-host disease. N Engl J Med 1992; 326: 105.

55. Parker P, Fahey JL, Schmidt GM et al. Thalidomide for the treatment of chronic graft-versus-host disease (GVHD). Blood 1989; 74; Suppl. 1: 123.

56. Hymes S, Morison WL, Farmer ER et al. Methoxypsoralen and ultraviolet A radiation in treatment of chronic cutaneous graft-versus-host reaction. Acad Dermatol 1985; 12: 30.

57. Atkinson K, Weller P, Ryman W et al. PUVA therapy for drug-resistant graft-versus-host disease. Bone Marrow Transplant 1990; 1: 227

58. Deeg H. Ultraviolet irradiation in transplantation biology. Manipulation of immunity and immunogenicity. Transplantation 1988; 45: 845.

59. Eppinger T, Ehninger G, Steinert M et al. 8-methoxypsoralen and ultraviolet A therapy for cutaneous manifestations of graft-versus-host disease. Transplantation 1990; 50: 807.

60. Kripke M. Immunological unresponsiveness induced by ultraviolet radiation. Immunol Rev 1984; 80: 87.

61. Bredberg A, Forsgren A. Effects of in vitro PUVA on human leukocyte function. Br J Dermatol 1984; 111: 159.

62. Granstein R, Lowy A, Greene M. Epidermal antigen-presenting cells in activation of suppression: Identification of a new functional type of ultraviolet radiation resistant epidermal cell. J Immunol 1985; 132: 563.

63. Okamoto H, Horio T, Meader M. Alteration of lymphocyte functions by 8 methoxypsoralen and long wave ultraviolet radiation. II. The effect of in vivo PUVA on IL-2 production. J Invest Dermatol 1987; 89: 24.

64. Kapoor N, Pelligrini AE, Copelan EA et al. Psoralen plus ultraviolet A (PUVA) in the treatment of chronic graft-versus-host disease: Preliminary experience in standard treatment resistant patients. Semin Hemat 1992; 29: 108.

65. van Prooijen H, Aarts-Riemens MI, Grijzenhout MA, van Weelden H. Ultraviolet irradiation modulates MHC-alloreactive cytotoxic T-cell precursors involved in the onset of graft-versus-host disease. Br J Haematol 1992; 81: 73.

66. Freid R, Murakami CS, Willson RA, Sullivan KM, McDonald GB. Chronic graft-vs-host disease of the liver: Another indication of ursodeoxycholic acid. Ann Intern Med 1992; 116: 233.

67. Eslinger S. Hepatology elsewhere. Hepatology 1992; 16: 1305.

68. Morris R, Meiser BM, Wu J et al. Use of rapamycin for the suppression of alloimmune reactions in vivo: Schedule-dependence, tolerance induction, synergy with cyclosporine and FK506 and effect on host-versus-graft and graft-versus-host reactions. Transplant Proc 1991; 23: 521.

69. Dumont F, Staruch MJ, Koprak SL et al. Distinct mechanisms of suppression of murine T-cell activation by the related macrolides FK-506 and rapamycin. J Immunol 1990; 144: 251.

70. Habeshaw J, Hounsell E, Dalgleish A. Does the HIV envelope induce a chronic graft-versus-host-like disease? Immunol Today 1992; 13: 207.

71. Simmonds P, Beatson D, Cuthbert R et al. Determinants of HIV disease progression: six year longitudinal study in Edinburgh haemophilia/HIV cohort. Lancet 1991; 338: 1159.

================CHAPTER 11================

# RELATED TOPICS

## GRAFT-VERSUS-LEUKEMIA EFFECT

Graft-derived cells exert an important part in the anti-leukemic effect.[1,2] This so-called graft-versus-leukemia (GVL) effect first became evident in comparing the different relapse rates among BMT patients with limited GVHD compared with those with more extensive chronic GVHD. The mechanisms and cell populations important in mediating graft-versus-leukemia are not completely understood. However, experimental and clinical data indicate that the immune-mediated GVL effect occurs following allogeneic bone marrow transplantation.[1,3] Potential cells involved in GVL include T cells which have been cloned (LAK cells and NK cells).[4,5] Other cytokines, such as IL-2, may enhance this anti-leukemic effect.[5] Clinically, it remains unclear whether GVL can be dissociated from GVHD. This is an important question since the GVL effect is a useful process that can decrease the relapse rate, whereas the graft-versus-host reaction can lead to an unwanted outcome. Thus, the optimal outcome would be to prevent GVHD without decreasing GVL. A murine leukemic and BMT model in which grafts of F1 hybrid origin are transplanted into parenteral strain animals was created to investigate GVL effects in a system that excludes graft-versus-host reactions. For genetic reasons, grafts of F1 hybrid origin are unable to induce an MHC-related graft-versus-host reaction in parental strain animals. The results suggest that there is a graft-versus-host reaction-independent GVL effect.[6] The death rate following transplantation of F1 marrow was significantly lower than after syngeneic transplantation. Depletion of Thy-1 cells from the bone marrow graft cause only a slight increase in the leukemic death rate after transplantation. Possible mechanism for a GVL effect independent of GVHD are reactions against antigens restricted to the hematopoietic system or specific cell types within the system. The anti-leukemic effect of semi-allogeneic bone marrow in the parental strain leukemia might be explained by the mechanism of natural resistance described for F1 hybrid animals receiving parental strain bone marrow. Thus, in murine models, this GVL effect can be separated from GVHD. It is also clear that these are murine models where the tumor is induced experimentally and not a naturally occurring disease. Such a model may not be directly applicable to the situation in humans. It remains unclear whether the same or different cell populations mediate the process of GVL and GVHD.

GVL clearly plays a very important role following allogeneic bone marrow transplantation in preventing or treating the recurrence of the underlying disease.[2] The best data to support this are comparisons of long-term, disease-free survival in patients transplanted for acute leukemia or receiving allogeneic bone marrow from matched sibling donors, compared to an identical sibling donor where the relapse rate is higher in the identical sibling donor. Recipients who develop GVHD have a lower incidence of leukemic relapse compared to those who do not develop GVHD.[1,3] The lowest rate of relapse occurs in patients with both acute and chronic GVHD. This GVL effect is further compounded by the use of immunosuppressive agents for the prevention of GVHD. Data suggest that cyclosporine can reduce the GVL effect in animal models and in patients.[7] This observation has also been extended to the clinical arena, where patients who receive cyclosporine for GVHD prophylaxis have a lower rate of GVHD but a higher relapse rate.[8]

The effect of cyclosporine A and methylprednisolone on the GVL effect across major MHC barriers in mice following allogeneic bone marrow transplantation has also been evaluated.[9] Using a murine model of originally spontaneous and subsequently transplantable nonimmunogenic B-cell leukemia (BCL1), investigators demonstrated that in mice treated with cyclosporine A, 89% of the mice developed leukemia within seven days. None of the methylprednisolone-treated mice or the untreated chimeras showed any evidence of leukemia for more than 150 days. This suggests that cyclosporine may impair the anti-leukemic effect exerted by allogeneic donor type immune cells against residual clonogenic leukemic cells which escape the chemoradiotherapy in tumor-bearing recipients. It is conceivable that different cells are responsible for GVHD and GVL. In the clinical trial using CD8 depletion only, data suggest that patients who receive a bone marrow depleted of CD8 cells only have a lower incidence of GVHD without a higher incidence of relapse, suggesting that the GVL effect was not decreased.[10-12]

## SYNGENEIC GVHD

Historically, GVHD is thought to be an allogeneic response of donor lymphocytes to the foreign histocompatibility antigen of the recipient. Several reports indicated that a GVH-like syndrome may occur after marrow transplantation performed between identical twins (syngeneic) or even after autologous BMT.[14,15] Various previous reports as early as the late 1950s and early 1960s defined a disease, termed isologous secondary disease, in mice surviving high lethal doses of TBI and rescue with small numbers of syngeneic bone marrow cells.[16,17] The histopathologic changes in these mice were similar to those seen with allogeneic GVHD, but generally were less severe. The histological analysis of the thymus showed an irreversible decrease in the numbers of epithelial cells in the thymus and may explain the occurrence of this isologous secondary disease (syngeneic GVHD).[18] As the secondary disease could be prevented by implantation of syngeneic newborn thymic fragments after the TBI and BMT, the initial evidence in these murine models suggests that thymic epithelial damage is a causative factor. A similar syndrome can also be observed in neonatal thymectomized mice.[19]

This observation has also been made in humans and a recent review has estimated that 10-15% of autologous or syngeneic BMT recipients develop this GVHD-like syndrome.[14] There has been a resurgence of interest in the experimental induction of syngeneic GVHD after autologous or syngeneic BMT.[20] Using a lethally irradiated rat model, investigators reconstituted these animals with syngeneic bone marrow and treated them with cyclosporine A for 40 days. The animals developed a T lymphocyte-dependent autoimmune syndrome 14 to 28 days after discontinuation of cyclosporine treatment. The syndrome appeared similar to that of GVHD. The T-cell response was directed against self-Ia antigens. In adoptive transfer experiments, large numbers of CD8 T cells from animals with syngeneic GVHD transferred a self-limited acute phase of the disease and the disease resolved within two weeks. Progression of the disease to a more chronic form of GVHD required the addition of CD4+ cells. In this rat model, the occurrence of syngeneic GVHD was dependent on treatment with cyclosporine for a minimum of 28 days. Shielding of the thymus during total body irradiation failed to induce this syndrome. The effect of cyclosporine on T-lymphocyte development has also been investigated in relationship to syngeneic GVHD.[21] Administration of cyclosporine following syngeneic BMT leads to the developmental arrest of mature CD4+ and CD8+ T lymphocytes in the thymus and a marked reduction in the cells expressing the $\alpha\beta$ T-cell receptor. Assessment of these cells revealed that CD8+ cells respond normally to mitogenic signaling whereas CD4+ cells exhibit marginal proliferative responses. T-cell differentiation in the thymus is rapidly restored to normal following the discontinuation of cyclosporine. A concurrent compensatory insurgence of CD4+ helper T cells is observed at the time of onset of syngeneic GVHD. These results suggest that ablation of lymphoid hematopoietic system is needed and that damage to the thymus is also needed to eliminate peripheral host auto regulatory mechanisms. The damaged thymus allows the egress of effector cells of syngeneic GVHD. Cyclosporine A appears to be important in augmenting development of autoreactive lymphocytes by blocking mechanisms that delete autoreactive T cells in the thymus.[22] Cyclosporine A is known to prevent the clonal deletion of MHC class II-restricted self-reactive T cells in the thymus.[23] Cyclosporine apparently inhibits thymocyte apoptosis induced by T-cell receptor signaling.[24] FK506 has also been used to induce pseudo-graft-versus-host disease or autologous GVHD similar to that induced by cyclosporine.[25]

Data also suggest that synergism exists with IL-2 and cyclosporine in inducing a GVL effect without GVHD following syngeneic BMT. When these two agents are combined, namely CsA and IL-2 following BMT, a potent GVL effect against melanoma and acute myelogenous leukemia is observed.[13] Adoptive transfer experiments into secondary recipients were successful in continuing this GVL effect. Cytotoxicity of these cells was not influenced by pretreatment of the tumor cells with interferon-γ or Ia antibody. The cytotoxic effect was mediated by Thy-1 and asialo GM-1 cells. These observations suggest the possibility of differences in the cellular mechanisms involved in GVL versus GVHD. This is an interesting combination in that cyclosporine may have induced a maturation arrest in T cells enough to break tolerance but not sufficient to cause overt GVHD.

The predominant interest in syngeneic GVHD is the possibility the effector T cells that mediate this auto-aggressive syndrome may be targeted to anti-tumor activity in the host. In animal models, the results suggest that syngeneic GVHD can mediate a significant anti-tumor effect achieving a 1-2 log tumor cell kill. Clinical studies aimed at exploiting this phenomena are ongoing.[26] Cutaneous GVHD was induced by the administration of cyclosporine to patients undergoing autologous BMT for AML.[26] Cyclosporine was administered for 28 days to 19 patients with AML who received busulfan, cyclophosphamide and autologous BMT with 4-hydroxy-peroxycyclophosphamide-treated marrow. It was a dose escalation trial where the cyclosporine doses were 1 mg/kg in seven patients, 2.5 mg/kg in eight patients or 3.75 mg /kg in four patients. Seventy-nine percent, or 15 of 19 patients, developed cutaneous histologic grade II GVHD at a median of 33 days. None developed any hepatic or GI dysfunction attributed to GVHD. Five patients with histopathologic grade II GVHD had no cutaneous changes observed clinically. The investigators concluded that they could induce acute GVHD after autologous BMT but did not observe any benefit for patients with positive biopsies in terms of reduced relapse rate or survival. A similar syndrome is observed in humans. Only long-term follow up in a prospective randomized trial will determine if there is clinical correlation with the occurrence of autologous GVHD and a decrease in the relapse rate.

There is some discrepancy with regard to the relationship of cyclosporine A-mediated inhibition of clonal deletion and the development of syngeneic GVHD. The idea that cyclosporine treatment may result in the inhibition of clonal deletion was tested by analyzing T-cell receptor expression as a measure of tolerance induction in a series of syngeneic radiation chimeras that were inducible and noninducible for syngeneic GVHD.[27] Clonal deletion assessed by anti-T-cell receptor Vβ chain monoclonal antibody occurred normally in strains of mice inducible for syngeneic GVHD. Conversely, animals in which T cells bearing self-reactive T-cell receptors could be detected did not develop syngeneic GVHD. Thus, the development of cyclosporine A induced autoreactive T cells as assessed by the Vβ T-cell receptor expression shows strain variation and does not correlate with the induction of syngeneic GVHD. These results suggest that other mechanisms may be involved in the development of this autoimmune phenomena.

The thymus has been studied following prolonged administration of cyclosporine.[28] The thymus shows irreversible changes associated with autologous GVHD. The immunopathologic changes seen in the thymus include medullary involution, loss of Hassall's corpuscles and decreased class II antigen expression. Generally, following short-term administration of cyclosporine, these changes are readily reversible. In rats, however, treated with mediastinal radiation, these changes become irreversible and are usually associated with changes of autologous or syngeneic GVHD. This is called pseudo-GVHD. Paralleling these thymic pathologic changes, acute and chronic pseudo-GVHD were observed in the skin, tongue, intestines, lacrimal glands, bronchi and intestines following long-term cyclosporine administration.

## TRANSFUSION-ASSOCIATED GVHD

The clinical scenario of GVHD may also occur in recipients of blood transfusions.[29] Transfused T cells can mediate transfusion-associated GVHD when given to patients with congenital immunodeficiency or patients who are undergoing high dose chemotherapy, radiation therapy or both.[30,31] Other patients such as those with Hodgkin's disease, who have deficits in T-cell function may also be at risk for transfusion-associated GVHD.[32] However, some patients with defects in cell-mediated immunity, such as patients with AIDS, appear not to be at risk for the disease. Finally, cases of transfusion-associated GVHD have also been reported in immunocompetent hosts.[33-35] Thus, the risk factors for the development of transfusion-associated GVHD remain poorly understood. Transfusion-associated GVHD is usually severe, frequently resulting in pancytopenia due to marrow aplasia. The majority of reported cases of transfusion-associated GVHD have been fatal, despite the use of immunosuppressive therapy. A comprehensive review of reported cases of transfusion-associated GVHD has been published.[36]

The first cases of transfusion-associated GVHD were reported in immunodeficient children after receiving transfusions. Exchange transfusion, intrauterine transfusion, as well as transfusion of whole blood, packed red cell buffy coats and granulocytes have been implicated in this phenomenon. The true incidence remains unknown, but is estimated to occur between 0.1-1% of patients with hematological cancers of lymphoproliferative diseases. The first case of transfusion-associated GVHD in a patient without obvious immune deficiency was reported in 1986.[33] This was a Japanese patient who survived surgery for an aortic aneurysm. A survey of 340 Japanese hospitals documented "postoperative erythroderma" in 24.5% of the patients who underwent cardiac surgery. The mortality rate was 90%.

The most commonly reported manifestations of transfusion-associated GVHD are rash, abnormal liver function tests and severe pancytopenia. There is an overall 84% mortality rate after a median 21 days of symptoms. There is no current evidence that any treatment for transfusion-associated GVHD influences the outcome. The cases of transfusion-associated GVHD reported after cardiac surgery in Japan occurred after transfusion of fresh whole blood. However, there is no evidence that avoiding transfusion of fresh blood products can prevent transfusion-associated GVHD. It is likely that the number of viable lymphocytes in the transfused product is more important. A comprehensive review by Greenbaum in 131 cases showed an overall 80% mortality in spite of treatment with immunosuppressive therapy. Not all cases of transfusion-associated GVHD manifest a complete clinical syndrome. Moreover, when these symptoms are present, it may be attributable to other etiologies such as infection or drug reaction. Therefore, it is likely that the true incidence of transfusion-associated GVHD is underreported. Since treatment is uniformly unsuccessful, the best method would be to prevent the occurrence of transfusion-associated GVHD. Methods to decrease the incidence of transfusion-associated GVHD include irradiation of the blood products by transfusion, filtration of the blood product, irradiation using gamma or UV irradiation. Although 15-20 Gy can reduce mitogen responsive lymphocytes by 5-6 logs, a small percentage of lymphocytes do survive radiation of these doses. There is a single reported case of apparent transfusion-associated GVHD in a BMT recipient who received only blood components irradiated at 20 Gy.

There are also multiple reports of transfusion-associated GVHD after transfusion of cellular blood components from donors homozygous for a given HLA haplotype to a first-degree family member who shares that haplotype.[37] This is a situation where the shared haplotype results in the lack of a host-versus-graft phenomena but the nonshared haplotype may allow for the expression of GVHD. It may be that extended haplotypes and the homogeneity in the Japanese population may make the occurrence of the transfusion-associated GVHD higher.

## GVHD FOLLOWING ORGAN TRANSPLANTATION

### LIVER

GVHD has been reported following organ transplantation. There is evidence that GVHD occurs after liver transplantation.[38] Not enough is known currently about the incidence, risk factors and mechanisms of GVHD in liver transplant recipients. Routine depletion of donor organ lymphocytes could be attempted, but could also result in adverse effects. Recent data suggests that limited donor engraftment with the establishment of a state of low-level mixed chimerism may promote acceptance of the organ.[39,40] Thus, if mixed chimerism is an important sequelae following solid organ transplantation, then depletion of donor lymphocytes could lead to increased incidence of organ rejection.

### KIDNEY

Bone marrow chimeras have been demonstrated with immune cytochemical and polymerase chain reaction techniques in kidney allografts and in the native skin, lymph nodes or blood in five of five patients who received continuously functioning renal transplants from one to two haplotype HLA-mismatched consanguineous donors.[41] These findings suggest that some migration, repopulation and chimerism are critical events that define graft acceptance and may ultimately lead to acquired donor-specific unresponsiveness or a state of tolerance.

### SMALL BOWEL

GVHD is a common problem following small bowel transplantation. The small bowel transplantation is capable not only of inducing graft-versus-host disease but also host-versus-graft reaction.[42] The severity of such immune responses is likely to be mediated by the large numbers of lymphoid cells in the mesenteric lymph nodes and Peyers' patches of the small intestine. Using UVB irradiation (700 J/M2) of bone marrow cells before transplantation into lethally irradiated allogeneic rats prevented GVHD and resulted in a stable chimerism. More importantly, this did not compromise bone marrow engraftment.

### REFERENCES

1. Weiden P, Flournoy MS, Thomas ED et al. Antileukemic effect of graft-versus-host disease in human recipients of allogeneic bone marrow transplantation. N Engl J Med 1979; 300: 1068.

2.  Kolb HJ, Mittermuller J, Clemm C et al. Donor leukocyte transfusions for treatment of recurrent chronic myelogenous leukemia in marrow transplant patients. Blood 1990; 76: 2462.

3.  Weiden P, Sullivan KM, Flournoy N et al. Anti-leukemic effect of chronic graft-versus-host disease: Contribution to improved survival after allogeneic marrow transplantation. N Engl J Med 1981; 304: 1529.

4.  Hauch M, Gazzola MV, Small T et al. Anti-leukemia potential of interleukin-2 activated natural killer cells after bone marrow transplantation for chronic myelogenous leukemia. Blood 1990; 75: 2250.

5.  Delmon L, Ythier A, Moingeon P et al. Characterization of anti-leukemia cells' cytotoxic effector function. Implications for monitoring natural killer responses following allogeneic bone marrow transplantation. Transplantation 1986; 42: 252.

6.  Glass B, Uharek L, Gassmann W et al. Graft-versus-leukemia activity after bone marrow transplantation does not require graft-versus-host disease. Ann Hematol 1992; 64: 255.

7.  Slavin S, Ackerstein A, Naparstek E et al. The graft-versus-leukemia (GVL) phenomenon: Is GVL separable from GVHD? Bone Marrow Transplant 1990; 6: 155.

8.  Barrett A, Horowitz MM, Gale RP et al. Marrow transplantation for acute lymphoblastic leukemia: Factors afffecting relapse and survival. Blood 1989; 74: 862.

9.  Weiss L, Reich S, Slavin S. Effect of cyclosporine A and methylprednisone on the graft-versus-leukemia effects across major histocompatibility barriers in mice following allogeneic bone marrow transplantation. Bone Marrow Transpl 1990; 6: 229.

10. Champlin R, Jansen J, Ho W et al. Retention of graft-versus-leukemia using selective depletion of CD8-positive T lymphocytes for prevention of graft-versus-host disease following bone marrow transplantation for chronic myelogenous leukemia. Transplant Proc 1991; 23: 1695.

11. Champlin R. Graft-versus-leukemia without graft-versus-host disease: An elusive goal of bone marrow transplantation. Semin Hemat 1992; 29: 46.

12. Champlin R, Ho W, Gajewski J et al. Selective depletion of CD8+ T lymphocytes for prevention of graft-versus-host disease after allogeneic bone marrow transplantation. Blood 1990; 76: 418.

13. Charak B, Agah R, Mazumder A. Synergism of interleukin-2 and cyclosporine A in induction of a graft-versus-host tumor effect without graft-versus-host disease after syngeneic bone marrow transplantation. Blood 1992; 80: 179.

14. Hood A, Vogelsang GB, Black LP, Farmer ER, Santos GW. Acute graft-versus-host disease: development following autologous and syngeneic bone marrow transplantation. Arch Dermatol 1987; 123: 745.

15. Rappeport J, Mihm M, Reinherz E, Lopansri S, Parkman R. Acute graft-versus-host disease in recipients of bone marrow transplants from identical twin donors. Lancet 1979; 2: 717.

16. van Bekkum D, Vos O, Weyzen WWH. The pathogenesis of the secondary disease after foreign bone marrow transplantation in x-irradiated mice. J Natl Cancer Inst 1959; 23: 75.

17. Barnes D, Ford CE, Ilbery PLT et al. Tissue transplantation in the radiation chimera. J Cell Comp Physiol 1957; 50(suppl 1): 123.

18. van Bekkum D. Immunological and hematological aspect of recovery: Implications for transplantation of bone marrow grafts. Brookhaven Symp Biol 1967; 20: 190.

19. van Bekkum D. Comments on syngeneic GVHD. Immunol Today 1990; 11: 107.

20. Glasier A, Tutschka PJ, Farmer ER, Santos GW. Graft-versus-host disease in cyclosporin A-treated rats after syngeneic and autologous bone marrow reconstitution. J Exp Med 1983; 158: 1.

21. Fischer A, Laulis MK, Horwitz L, Hess AD. Effect of cyclosporine on T lymphocyte development. Transplantation 1991; 51: 252.

22. Beschorner W, Ren H, Phillips J, Pulido H, Hruban RH, Hess AD. Prevention of syngeneic graft-versus-host- disease by recovery of thymic microenvironment after cyclosporine. Transplantation 1991; 5: 668.

23. Jenkins M, Schwartz RH, Pardoll DM. Effects of cyclosporine A on T-cell development and clonal deletion. Science 1988; 241: 1655.

24. Shi Y, Sahai BM, Green DR. Cyclosporine A inhibits activation-induced cell death in T-cell hybridomas and thymocytes. Nature 1989; 339: 625.

25. Cooper M, Hartman GG, Starzl TE, Fung JJ. The induction of pseudo-graft-versus-host disease following syngeneic bone marrow transplantation using FK 506. Transplant Proc 1991; 23: 3234.

26. Yeager A, Vogelsang GB, Jones RJ et al. Induction of cutaneous graft-versus-host disease by administration of cyclosporine to patients undergoing autologous bone marrow transplantation for acute myeloid leukemia. Blood 1992; 79: 3031.

27. Bryson J, Caywood BE, Kaplan AM. Relationship of cyclosporine A-mediated inhibition of clonal deletion and development of syngeneic graft-versus-host disease. J Immunol 1991; 147: 391.

28. Shinozawa T, Beschorner WE, Hess AD. The thymus and prolonged administration of cyclosporine. Transplantation 1990; 50: 106.

29. Anderson K, Weinstein HJ. Transfusion-associated graft-versus-host disease. N Engl J Med 1990; 323: 315.

30. Armitage R, Goldstone AH, Richards JD, Cawley JC. Lymphocyte function after autologous bone marrow transplantation (BMT): A comparison with patients treated with allogeneic BMT and with chemotherapy only. Br Med J 1986; 63: 637.

31. Reinherz E, Geha R, Pappeport JM et al. Reconstitution after transplantation with T-lymphocyte-depleted HLA haplotype-mismatched bone marrow for severe combined immunodeficiency. Proc Natl Acad Sci USA 1982; 79: 6047.

32. Twomey J, Rice L. Impact of Hodgkin's disease upon the immune system. Semin Oncol 1980; 7: 114.

33. Sakakibara T, Juji T. Post-transfusion graft-versus-host disease after open heart surgery. Lancet 1986; 2: 1099.

34. Vogelsang G. Transfusion-associated graft-versus-host disease in nonimmunocompromised hosts. Transfusion 1990; 30: 101.

35. Arsura L, Bertelle A, Minkowitz S, Cunningham JN Jr, Grob D. Transfusion-associated graft-vs-host disease in a presumed immunocompetent patient. Arch Intern Med 1988; 148: 1941.

36. Greenbaum B. Transfusion-associated graft-versus-host disease: Historical perspectives, incidence, and current use of irradiated blood products. J Clin Oncol 1991; 9: 1889.

37. Thaler M, Shamiss A, Orgad S et al. The role of blood from HLA-homozygous donors in fatal transfusion-associated graft-versus-host disease after open heart surgery. N Engl J Med 1989; 321: 25.

38. DePaoli A, Bitran J. Graft-versus-host disease and liver transplantation. Ann Int Med 1992; 117: 170.

39. Collins R, Cooper C, Nikaein A, Klintmalm G, Fay J. Graft-versus-host disease in a liver transplant recipient. Ann Intern Med 1992; 116: 391.

40. Starzl TE, Demetris AJ, Trucco M et al. Chimerism after liver transplantation for type IV glycogen storage disease and type I Gaucher's disease. N Engl J Med 1993; 28: 745.

41. Starzl TE, Demetris AJ, Trucco M et al. Chimerism and donor-specific nonreactivity 27 to 29 years after kidney allotransplantation. Transplantation 1993; 55: 1272.

42. Kirkham R. Small bowel transplantation. Transplantation 1984; 37: 429.

# CHAPTER 12

# CONCLUSION

Knowledge accumulated over the past 70 years beginning with an observation in chicken embryos has led to successful allogeneic bone marrow transplantation in humans. Much of the preliminary work focused on understanding whether a specific cell type was involved. Today, it is clear that T cells are important in the establishment of GVHD.

Most of the current clinical data have focused on methods to prevent GVHD. As with any disease, prevention is the best method. The most common form is to use immunosuppressive drugs to achieve prophylaxis. The second most common approach of immunosuppression is to deplete the T cells that cause the disease. Many trials have been conducted to treat GVHD and, to date, most of the data suggest that once GVHD occurs, there is only limited success with such approaches.

The future for the prevention of GVHD will continue to parallel our understanding of immunology and molecular biology. These approaches include the following:

1. prevention of peptide binding to the MHC molecules
2. manipulation of the secondary signal by interfering with B7-2
3. attenuation of the cytokine response by interfering with IL-1, IL-2, interferon-$\gamma$, TNF, etc
4. manipulation of the T-cell subsets such as selective T-cell depletion
5. skewing of the T-cell repertoire towards $T_h2$ versus $T_h1$ cells
6. insertion of recipient MHC genes the donor cells
7. and possibly, infusion of pure populations of hematopoietic stem cells from allogeneic donors or fetal cord blood cells

Individually or in combination, these approaches will lead to safer allogeneic BMT. At the same time, there is the need to preserve the graft-versus-leukemia effect since this form of immunomodulation is also important in the ultimate outcome of the patient. The plethora of possibilities for the prevention of GVHD in the future make this indeed an exciting field.

# INDEX

*Items in italics denote figures (f) or tables (t).*